PATHOPHYSIOLOGY AND CLINICAL ASPECTS OF VENOUS THROMBOEMBOLISM IN NEONATES, RENAL DISEASE AND CANCER PATIENTS

Edited by **Mohammed A. Abdelaal**

Pathophysiology and Clinical Aspects of Venous Thromboembolism in Neonates, Renal Disease and Cancer Patients
Edited by Mohammed A. Abdelaal

Published by InTech

Janeza Trdine 9, 51000 Rijeka, Croatia

Publishing Process Manager Dejan Grgur

Technical Editor Teodora Smiljanic

Cover Designer InTech Design Team

Additional hard copies can be obtained from orders@intechopen.com

Pathophysiology and Clinical Aspects of Venous Thromboembolism in Neonates, Renal Disease and Cancer Patients, Edited by Mohammed A. Abdelaal
p. cm.
ISBN 978-953-51-0616-6

Meet the editor

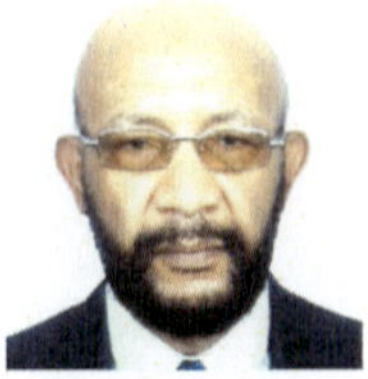

Dr Mohamed A. Abdelaal, MD, FRCPath, FRCPI, is a senior Consultant Hematologist at the Adult Hematology/Adult BMT, Princess Noorah Oncology Center, King Abdulaziz Medical City, Jeddah, Saudi Arabia. He trained in hematology at the Hammersmith Hospital and the London Hospital in Whitechapel, UK, before he took up his current position in 1987. In addition, Dr Abdelaal holds the position of Chairman of Pathology and Laboratory Medicine, and Head of King Abdullah International Medical Research Center. Dr Abdelaal holds several achievement awards and is very active on various fronts of teaching, academics, and research with over 90 publications, management, quality improvement and auditing. His areas of research interest are thromboembolism, leukemia and lymphoma.

Contents

Preface

The estimated total number of symptomatic venous thromboembolism (VTE) events per annum within six European communities was 465,715 cases of DVT; 295,982 cases of PE and 370,012 VTE related deaths and almost three quarters of all VTE-related deaths were hospital–acquired deaths.

Across the Atlantic, VTE is a major health problem in the USA with the annual incidence of VTE of 108 per 100,000 person/year among Caucasians, with 250,000 incident cases occurring annually among the Caucasians in the United States. Among African Americans, the incidence appears to be similar or higher, but among the Asian and native-Americans, the incidence is lower.

In the Far East, VTE is not as common in Chinese as in Caucasians but is certainly not rare. The incidence of DVT and PE was reported to the 17.1 and 3.9 per 100,000 populations, respectively.

Understanding the etiology and pathogenesis of thrombosis is important for developing management strategy including preventive. In this book, we have selected two important etiological aspects of venous thrombosis to highlight microparticles and homocysteine. Flowcytometry has shown that the levels of platelet-derived microparticles and endothelial-derived microparticles to be elevated in deep vein thrombosis and cardiovascular disease can constitute to hypercoagulability due to circulating procoagulant microparticles. To that end, Dr. Enjeti from Australia assembled a very informative account, chapter 1, on the role of microparticles in hemostasis and venous thromboembolism and concluded that there are three potential areas where measuring the microparticles with respect to VTE may be relevant: diagnostic, prognostic and therapeutic.

Hyperhomocysteinemia is a known risk factor for VTE. The risk of VTE recurrence in patients with hyperhomocysteinemia is unknown and so is the management of those patients after acute event of VTE. Dr. Plazar and Dr. Jurdana from Slovenia, Chapter 2, present a detailed updated account on this important topic including diagnosis and management.

VTE is an important clinical problem because of the associated morbidity and mortality and its negative impact on the Healthcare System. The medical literature is very rich in publications on the subject, epidemiology, etiology, pathogenesis, risk stratification, VTE in different groups of medical and surgical conditions, diagnosis, management, guidelines for thromboprophylaxis and management. As it is not possible to have a comprehensive book that covers all aspects of VTE, in this book we have elected to address certain etiological aspects of venous thrombosis: VTE in neonates, children, chronic renal disease and VTE in cancer patient with special reference to anti-cancer agents associated with high risk of VTE, especially in tertiary care settings.

Several national and international registries have helped to define the epidemiology, risk factors for VTE in different age groups and demonstrated the important differences between VTE in adults and pediatric patients and called for evidence-based guidelines for management and prevention of VTE in neonates and children. In chapter 3, Dr. Lazaro and colleagues described the magnitude of this problem including diagnosis and management.

The same authors also gave a detailed account of VTE in patients with chronic renal disease, with special reference to epidemiology, pathogenesis, and treatment in this important group of patients with a special reference to unfractionated heparin, low molecular heparin, the pentasaccharide and some of the novel oral anticoagulants.

Although cancer has been clearly associated with venous thromboembolism, many aspects of this relation are still not well understood, including the cancer sites most associated with VTE and the risk for cancer development during follow-up of patients with idiopathic VTE. In chapter 4, the authors have depicted an informative updated account on the epidemiology, pathogenesis, patient-related factors, cancer-related factors and treatment related factors and their impact on the risk of VTE in cancer patients with special emphasis on some chemotherapeutic agents associated with VTE. The authors also put up some practical information on thromboprophylaxis in cancer patients at different clinical settings.

The use of immunomodulatory agents thalidomide and, lately, its second generation Lenalidomide, has revolutionized the management of multiple myeloma patients. However, their use carries a significant risk of thrombosis. Dr. Mateos and Dr. Gonzalez-Porras, chapter 5, assembled an excellent account on those agents in a practical format, which helps the practicing oncologists and hematologists in handling those effective agents to minimize the risk of the VTE associated with the use of those agents.

Dr. Agutter and Dr. Malone from Theoretical Medicine and Biology Group, UK, argued elegantly for a rational approach for mechanical thromboprophylaxis in chapter 6. The authors summarized the valve cusp hypoxia hypothesis, discussed its clinical implications and suggested a sound approach to prophylaxis based on this hypothesis.

In their descriptive account in Chapter 7, titled Venous Thromboembolism as a Preventable Patient Injury - Experience of the Danish Patient Insurance Association

(1996 - 2010), Dr. Christoffersen and Dr. Hove describe situations where VTE may be judged to be a patient injury and the cases cited from the database all emphasize the need for healthcare practitioner to be aware of the medico-legal aspects of VTE cases, and use updated approved guidelines on VTE prophylaxis.

The medical practice guidelines are usually prepared by standing Task Force/Committees and approved by Executive and/or Council. These evidence-based guidelines reflect emerging clinical and scientific advances in the specific clinical discipline and related specialties as to the date of issue. However, they are subject to change and local institutions are advised that they may modify the guidelines for their own use with full documentation of those modifications. Moreover, the guideline are not meant as dictating an exclusive line of treatment or procedure to be followed and are not intended to substitute the clinical judgment of the attending physician.

The American Public Health Association issued a white paper in 2003, entitled "Deep Vein Thrombosis: Awareness to protect patient lives" and issued a call for action stating that DVT and PE constitute major health problem in the USA and more people die of PE than motor vehicle accidents, breast cancer or AIDS, and physicians, healthcare providers, public heath advocates and consumers must be aware of the preventability of this epidemic and act accordingly.

For patients with a high/very high risk of VTE combined pharmacological and mechanical prophylaxis should be ordered. However, failure of physicians and healthcare providers to adhere to VTE prophylaxis guidelines/protocols in high/very high-risk patients remains a problem in many countries. Hospitals with adequate electronic information systems may consider implementation of electronic alerts to enforce adherence to thromboprophylaxis guidelines/protocols. However, the same strategy can be implemented by institutions without electronic systems if the awareness and willingness of the healthcare providers to cooperate on this important aspect of patient's safety is ensured. In the near future, the voluntary aspects of ordering thromboprophylaxis is very likely to be replaced with an obligatory one, as regulating authorities and insurance companies demand that VTE is a preventable patient injury.

Dr Mohamed A. Abdelaal
Senior Consultant Hematologist, Head of Pathology & Laboratory Medicine;
Head of King Abdullah International Medical Research Center
Jeddah, Saudi Arabia

Section 1

Some Aspects of Pathogenesis of Thrombosis

1

Microparticles: Role in Haemostasis and Venous Thromboembolism

Anoop K. Enjeti[1] and Michael Seldon[2]
[1,2]*Calvary Mater and John Hunter Hospitals, University of Newcastle,*
[2]*Hunter Area Pathology Service,*
Australia

1. Introduction

Microparticles (MP) are small membrane bound vesicles which have been described in circulation. They are derived from a variety of cells by an active process of shedding. They are bound by plasma membrane, are anucleate but may contain DNA or RNA and may be virtually derived from any cell (Ahn 2005, Mause, *et al*, Porto, *et al*). The majority of the microparticles in blood are derived from platelets. Previously considered as cell debris they are now regarded as vectors for transfer of biological information. The MP production is thought to reflect a balance between cell stimulation, proliferation and death. Based on their potential function and pathophysiologic effect, MP are thought to be physiological or patholological. MP play a role in normal haemostasis and abnormal amplification of MP production leading to a pathological state (Meziani, *et al*). For example, excessive MP from platelets may contribute to thrombosis (Siljander, *et al* 1996). Their role in vascular biology is being uncovered with increasing evidence for their role in venous thromboembolism. This chapter will explore the role of these MP in the physiology of haemostasis as well as pathology of thromboembolism. The final section will discuss the current state of art in the methods used to detect and measure MP.

1.1 Definition of a microparticle

Microparticles are submicron (<1.0µm) membrane bound circulating vesicles. Although anucleate, usually express cell surface antigen specific to the cell of origin, they may contain DNA or RNA and be virtually derived from any cell (Freyssinet 2003). The ISTH (International Society of Thrombosis and Haemostasis) vascular biology subcommittee defined these particles as being between 0.1-1.0 µm (SSCMembers Aug 2005). However, several other nanoscale techniques have demonstrated that particles <0.1 µm may also need to be considered as MP (Yuana, *et al*). Indeed, size range of MP is contentious with larger MP likely overlapping with small platelets and the smallest MP with exosomes (Gyorgy, *et al*, Jy, *et al*, Lawrie, *et al* 2009). Several factors may cause the production of MP from cells such as activation, complement mediated lysis, shearing stress, oxidative injury and active vesiculation (Horstman, *et al* 2004). The MP bear at least some surface characteristics of the parent cell and they differ from exosomes (0.03-0.1µm), which originate through the exocytosis of endocytic multivesicular bodies and play a role in antigen presentation (Freyssinet and Dignat-George 2005, Horstman, *et al* 2004, Horstman, *et al* 2007).

Cellular source of MPs	Marker	Proportion in circulation
Platelets	CD61 (GPIIIa) CD63 CD62p (P-selectin) CD41	80-90%
Leucocytes	CD45	<5%
Erythrocytes	Glycophorin A	5-10%
T helper cells	CD4	<1%
T cytotoxic cells	CD8	<1%
B cells	CD20	<1%
Monocytes/ macrophages	CD14	<5%
Endothelial cells	CD62e (E-selectin)	<5%

Table 1. Microparticle source, surface antigen expression and proportion in circulation (Enjeti, *et al* 2007, Siljander).

2. Microparticles: Production and role in haemostasis

2.1 How are microparticles produced?

Microparticles are thought to be produced by an active process of vesiculation or shedding from the cell surface and utilizing ATP in the process. Various enzymes involved in the production of MP have been studied. The balance of several enzymes regulating membrane homeostasis is believed to be key in the production of MP. An inward aminophospholipid enzyme 'translocase' or 'flippase'and an outward enzyme 'floppase' have been postulated to maintain the dynamic symmetrical state of the phophoslipid bilayer membrane (Diaz and Schroit 1996, Montoro-Garcia, *et al*, Morel, *et al*). In a resting membrane the flippase enzyme is more active thereby ensuring that phosphotidyl serine (PS) is at the inner membrane.The activation of phospholipid nonspecific enzyme known as 'scramblase' is said to be responsible for disruption of membrane asymmetry and several mechanisms participating in the regulation of the transmembrane migration of phosphatidylserine (PS) in activated cells lead to microparticle shedding (Diaz and Schroit 1996, Enjeti, *et al* 2008, Morel, *et al* 2006). After stimulation, calcium is released from intracellular stores. Calcium depletion induces the activation of store-operated calcium entry (SOCE) through channels in the plasma membrane and this process is thought to be regulated by transient receptor potential channel (TRPC) proteins (Diaz and Schroit 1996, Montoro-Garcia, *et al*). The transverse redistribution of PS is under the control of SOCE. Several other process such as Raft integrity, cytoskeleton organization and MAP kinase pathway (Ras-ERK) are also involved in membrane remodelling (Diaz and Schroit 1996, Montoro-Garcia, *et al*, Morel, *et al* 2006). Microparticles typically have phosphotidyl serine on the outer surface (although PS negative MP have also been recently described) and ABCA1, a member of the ATP-binding cassette family of transporters, is a potential candidate for the transport of PS to the surface (Diaz and Schroit 1996, Morel, *et al* 2006).

2.2 Role of MP in coagulation and haemostasis

Normal coagulation is a complex process triggered by endothelial damage and exposure of tissue factor and collagen which initiates a platelet plug formation at the site of injury. This leads to activation of a cascade of enzymes, which forms a fibrin clot. Microparticles of different cell origin could play a role in fibrin clot formation, enhance platelet leukocyte interactions and influence other plasma proteins such as von Willebrand's factor. Given that platelet MP constitute the majority of the circulating MP, they are considered an important effector of the haemostatic process (Morel, *et al* 2006). Some MP have also been described to carry molecules with anticoagulant function on their surface (Freyssinet 2003). The balance of pro and anticoagulant bearing MP in the endovascular milieu is likely to influence the propensity to bleed or clot in a particular patient.

Type of MP	Example of surface marker on MP
Procoagulant	von Willebrand's Factor Tissue Factor Platelet Factor 3 activity
Anti-coagulant	Tissue Factor Pathway inhibitor Protein C/S Thrombomodulin

Table 2. The possible pro and anticoagulant markers on the surface of microparticles (Enjeti, *et al* 2007, Morel, *et al* 2006).

2.3 Platelet MP

2.3.1 Platelet MP and coagulation

Traditionally, platelets major function was thought to be due to their aggregability and ability to plug damaged endothelium and capillary vessels. More recently, they are thought to form an important substrate for the coagulation pathway with their membrane providing the surface for the formation of the prothrombinase complex (comprising the Xa and Va complex). This enzyme complex leads to conversion of fibrinogen to fibrin which in combination with a variety of other factors leads to a stable clot at the site of injury. The presence of platelet microparticles at the site of blood vessel injury may contribute to this process by providing a large source of surface membrane for assembly of the enzymatic process. Indeed the exposure of phosphotidylserine at the site of thrombin generation increases the enzymatic catalyic effect by several hundred fold (Aleman). Platelets thus appear to have two major physiological roles for achieving haemostasis - form a platelet plug at the site of endothelial injury and generate microparticles which provide a surface for activation of the coagulation cascade leading to formation of the fibrin clot. The third possible role for the platelet MP could possibly be in maintaining the integrity of normal resting endothelium (Cambien, 2004). This area is still being actively explored. The role of MP in haemostasis is illustrated in figure 1.

Apart from procoagulant function MP could also be involved in anticoagulant activity. Microparticles with TFPI (tissue factor pathway inhibitor) and antithrombin activity have been described (Morel, *et al* 2006, Siljander). However, the anticoagulant MP have not been as extensively studied and it would be interesting to evaluate these MP - its association with pathologic conditions.

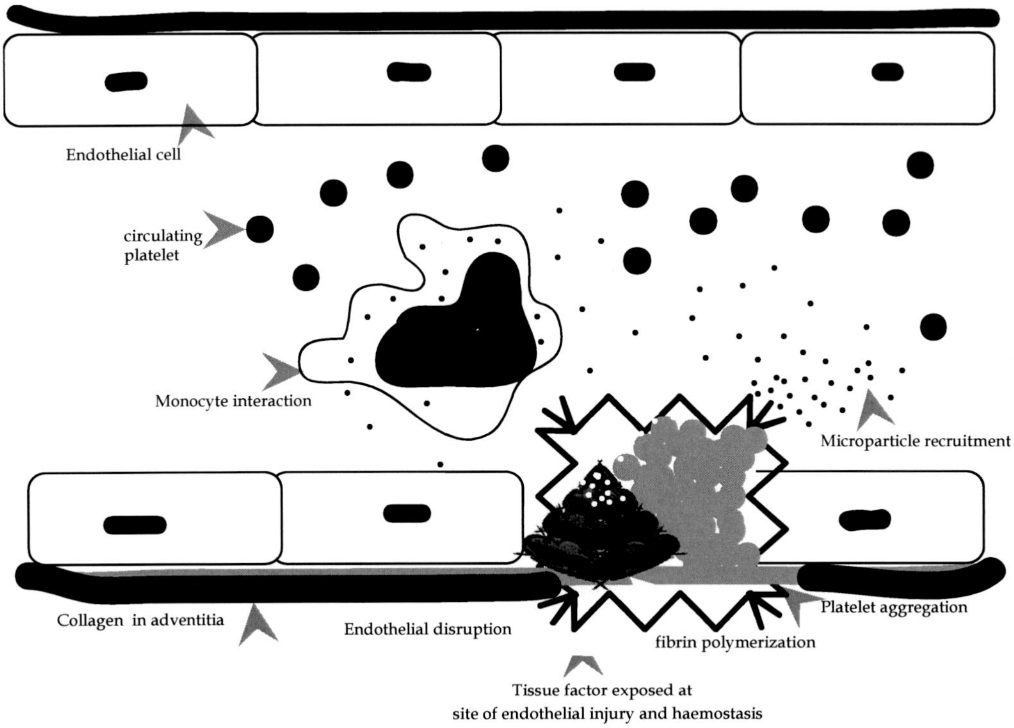

Fig. 1. The interaction of MP of platelet and monocyte origin being recruited in thrombus formation at site of endothelial injury.

2.3.2 Molecular interactions of Platelet MP

Platelet MP also bear a number of antigens such GPIIbIIIa, GPIa, von Willebrand's factor and arachidonic acid which may all be important effectors in the clotting mechanism. The understanding of the molecular mechanisms of haemostasis has now led to the thinking that coagulation can be described as an interaction between p-selection, tissue factor thrombin and microparticles (Furie and Furie 2004). P-selectin is an adhesion molecule expressed at the platelet endothelial interface which is thought to be critical for tissue factor activity and leukocyte adhesion in the thrombus (Myers, 2003). Some authors have even described P-selectin on microparticles, tissue factor and clotting proteins as being the molecular triad for coagulation (Polgar, 2005).

Another potential role of MP may be in the interaction of endothelium, von Willebrand's factor and platelets.The platelet derived microparticles could interact with the protease ADAMTS-13 (**A** **D**isintegrin **A**nd **M**etalloproteinase with **T**hrombo**S**pondin-1-like motifs, member **13** of this family of metalloprotease) , which regulates the activity of high molecular weight von Willebrand's factor. Increased microparticles in circulation could potentially compete in binding ADAMTS-13, reducing its interaction with the endothelium and influencing multimer cleavage (Jy, *et al* 2005). This may then contribute to the increased rates of thrombosis observed in these patients with thrombotic thrombocytopaenic purpura though the evidence for this process is very preliminary.

2.4 Tissue factor bearing MP

In an intact blood vessel tissue factor is usually restricted to adventitia and protected by the endothelial layer. However, small amounts of monocyte related tissue factor have been isolated in circulation (Key). The presence of tissue factor (TF) bearing microparticles, mainly derived from monocytes, in circulation has been shown to participate in initiation of fibrin polymerization (Eilertsen and Osterud 2004, Key). Although usually found to be in very small numbers in normal circulation, these increase dramatically at the site of injury. The interaction between tissue factor bearing MP and platelet MP is also of interest as there appears to be some evidence that they may be complementary in terms of thrombin generation potential (Key and Kwaan).

2.5 Modelling MP in thrombosis

The evidence for the involvement of these MP in its various physiological roles in haemostasis comes from the following models.

2.5.1 Cell based haemostasis model

The initial evidence for the role of MP in haemostasis comes from the cell based model. In this model plasma coagulation proteins are activated on the membrane surface after exposure to tissue factor. This leads to enzymatic cleavage of thrombin from prothrombin which ultimately converts fibrinogen to fibrin. This forms the fibrin clot and leads to haemostasis along with other components of the clot such as platelets and monocytes (Biro, *et al* 2003, Chirinos, *et al* 2005).

2.5.2 Live imaging model

Studies using intravital microscopy have shown that TF bearing MP derived from haemopoietic cells are incorporated into a thrombus. A laser injury model using the cremaster muscle arterioles of the mouse showed that MP participate in thrombosis (Falati, *et al* 2003). Although these studies visualize incorporation of TF bearing MP into the thrombus, it is not yet known if these MP are actually functional.

2.5.3 Animal models

These studies have involved introducing exogenous MP from patients or other source into animal models. In one such study MP from patients with acute coronary syndrome were introduced in to a rat model triggered venous thrombosis (Mallat, *et al* 2000). This study supports the role of TF bearing MP in promotion of VTE, However, the cellular sources of this TF has not been entirely clarified in other studies (Shantsila, *et al*).

2.5.4 Scott Syndrome

Scott Syndrome is an extremely rare hemorrhagic disorder characterized by bleeding diathesis (only three well documented cases of Scott syndrome have been reported to date) (Zwaal, *et al* 2004). The bleeding tendency is thought to be due to impaired procoagulant activity of stimulated platelets - the platelets being unable to expose anionic phospholipids and to shed procoagulant microparticles. The exposure of the aminophospholipids, mainly phosphatidylserine, on surface of stimulated platelets or derived microparticles, is critical for the formation of enzyme complexes in the clotting process (Zwaal, *et al* 2004, Zwaal, *et al* 2005). Mutations involving the ABCA1 ATP transporter have been reported in this syndrome (Zwaal, *et al* 2004).

There are several other mechanisms by which MP influence the endovascular system. They may modulate endothelial function and carry proangiogeneic molecules (Lozito and Tuan). Recently MP bearing Sonic hedgehog have been shown modulate angiogenesis (Soleti, *et al* 2009, Soleti and Martinez 2009). They may also serve as novel carriers for transport of genetic material - such as mRNA or microRNA and these are currently areas of intense research (Rak).

3. Role in thrombosis

From their role in physiology of haemostasis it can be extrapolated that excess production of MP will lead to a pathological state. Indeed, increase in circulating MP have been described in a wide variety of states. The role of MP in various thrombotic states is discussed below.

3.1 Venous Thromboembolism (VTE)

3.1.1 Idiopathic VTE

Venous thromboembolism is the result of a complex interaction between the circulating proteins, cells/platelets and the endothelium (Collen and Hoylaerts 2005). There is no known provoking or identifiable precipitating factor in idiopathic VTE. A recent study looked at the interactions between the MP of various origin - platelet, endothelial and monocyte and endothelial derived MPs were found to be elevated in association with VTE. One report suggests that the combination of total circulating MP, P-selectin levels and D-dimer levels may help predict VTE (Rectenwald, *et al* 2005). This approach had a sensitivity of 73% indicating the need for further refinement for application in clinical practise.

In another larger investigation no association was found between levels of total circulating MP and risk of recurrent VTE (Ay, *et al* 2009). Interestingly, a study comparing patients with cancer who had VTE and those with idiopathic VTE found raised tissue factor bearing MP only in cancer patients (Thaler, *et al*). In another report, plasma levels of tissue factor MP were not raised in those with pulmonary embolism suggesting that that perhaps other subtypes of MP may have to be studied in more detail to explain the relationship found in experimental models (Garcia Rodriguez, *et al* 2010). Owen and co authors looked at the recurrence of VTE and found that the procoagulant activity but not number of MP was increased in cases of recurrence (Owen, *et al*).

The role of MP in predicting thrombosis in those with heritable thrombophilia has also been explored. It has been found that total circulating MP levels were increased in subjects with heterozygote factor V Leiden status but there was no difference between those who had had VTE and those without (Enjeti, *et al* 2010). This finding and other studies seems to suggest that although total microparticles have been shown to be increased in those with VTE or those prone for VTE, there appears to be no convincing data that MP help to predict or monitor VTE. However, in a recent study that investigated this issue further, looked at MP levels by a different approach by comparing percentiles of MP measured in a retrospective case-control fashion. In those with circulating MP above the 90th percentile of the control population's distribution, a five fold increased risk was observed (Bucciarelli, 2011). They found that elevated MP were indeed an independent risk factor for VTE and this warrants a confirmation in a prospective cohort study.

The draw back of the studies in this area of VTE include the variability of type of MP studied, the techniques employed for measurement of MP and retrospective nature of investigations undertaken.

3.1.2 Immune related VTE

In contrast to idiopathic VTE, there is strong evidence for involvement of MP in thrombogeneticity in patients with underlying immune disorders. Important examples include antiphospholipid antibody syndrome and heparin induced thrombocytopaenia with thrombosis syndromes (Combes, *et al* 1999, Dignat-George, *et al* 2004, Walenga, *et al* 2000). Markedly elevated platelet derived MP have been desccribed in both clinical syndromes (Hughes, 2000). There is experimental evidence to suggest that circulating autoantibodies trigger the formation of excess MP contributing to the prothrombotic process in these patients. Circulating MP in these syndromes have been shown to expose GPIb,GPIIbIIIa, P-selectin and thrombospondin all of which help promote thrombosis (Jy, *et al* 2007).

3.1.3 Microparticles, VTE and cancer

In contrast to the above discussion for idiopathic VTE - thrombosis, cancer and microparticles seem to have a more definitive relationship. The MP are thought to reflect a balance between cell stimulation, proliferation and death which may be important in cancer related thrombosis. Cancer increases the risk of VTE by four fold and addition of chemotherapy further increases the risk by six to eight fold (Furie and Furie 2006). It is possible that circulating MP shed from cancer cells represent an indication for tumours to metastasize in the absence of any other clinical evidence for metastasis. A recent report states that platelet MP markedly stimulated the metastatic potential of 5 different cancer cell lines (Rak). It has also been shown that human tumor derived MP when injected into mice activated coagulation by virtue of their TF procoagulant activity (Thaler).

Procoagulant properties of tumor cell MP have been an area of intense study. A range of endothelial, monocyte and leukocyte MP along with tissue factor bearing MP appear to have a coagulant potential and have shown to be elevated in various such as cancers such as pancreatic, breast and prostate (Pilzer, *et al* 2005, Simak and Gelderman 2006).

A recent in vivo live microscopy mouse model with pancreatic cancer demonstrated that TF bearing MP released from the cancer cells entered circulation and participated in the thrombus formation at a distant site (Thomas, 2009).

The most important evidence for role of MP in VTE and cancer comes from clinical studies showing increased numbers and procoagulant activity of MP in cancer (Langer). Elevated levels of tissue factor bearing MP were associated with VTE events in those with advanced malignancy particularly pancreatic cancer. The microparticle levels in cancer patients also predicted the development of thrombosis, with the one year estimate of those with TF bearing MP being about 34% (Thaler, 2011). In contrast those who did not develop thrombosis did not have a detectable level of tissue factor bearing microparticles.

3.1.4 Disease groups associated with venous or arterial thrombosis

There are a number of conditions associated with elevated MP. Most of these disease states are associated with an increased risk of thrombosis. They essentially seem to reflect the health and pathophysiology of the endovascular system. Table 3 below gives a list of conditions where they have been found to be elevated.

Condition	Specific example where MP were elevated (reference)
Cardiovascular disease	Hypertension (Boulanger) Myocardial infarct/angina (Nagy) (Exner, 2005) Stroke (Merten, 2004) Diabetes (Alkhatatbeh) Thromboembolism (Cimmino)
Myeloproliferative Disorder	Polycythemia vera (Duchemin) Essential Thrombocytosis (Villmow, 2002) Myelofibrosis (Villmow, 2002)
Thrombotic Microangiopathies	Thrombotic thrombocytopaenic purpura (Ahn, 2002) Pre-eclampsia of pregnancy (Aharon)
Autoimmune diseases	Antiphopholipid antibody syndrome (Combes, 1999;Dignat-George, 2004) Systemic lupus erythematosis (Nielsen; Pereira, 2006)
Cancer related	Metastatic solid tumours (Dass, 2007) Chemotherapy induced (Kim, 2002; Kim) Neoangiogenesis (Goon, 2006)

Table 3. List of conditions associated with thrombosis and elevated MPs in circulation.

3.2 Microparticles and atherothrombosis

The role of MP in promoting atherothrombosis has also been another area of study (Cimmino). In one report, shed membrane microparticles were seen to be produced in human atherosclerotic plaques and were a critical determinant of thrombogenecity after plaque rupture (Mallat, 1999). The apoptosis occurring after plaque disruption or rupture was closely associated with TF expression on cell membranes leading to thrombogenecity. These MP were observed to express phosphotidylserine and some expressed CD11a which is an adhesion molecule (Martinez, 2005) (Morel, 2006). Given the links between inflammation and thrombosis, the emerging role of MP in atherothrombosis is not surprising (McGregor, 2006; Meerarani, 2007).

4. Measuring microparticles

There are several approaches to detection and measurement of MP. The methods are usually based on the ability of the assay to either enumerate or assess functional activity of the MP.

4.1 Functional assays

Most of the assays under this section relate to either the prothrombotic function of MP or measuring the phospholipid content of MP. This can be done in the liquid phase e.g. a clot based assay such as the XACT test or by estimation of prothrombinase activity using an ELISA (Exner, 2003). The advantages of these approaches are that they provide an indication of the procoagulant activity of MP. The drawback is that the cell of origin for the MP cannot be determined.

4.2 Quantitative assays

Flow cytometry is the most widely employed quantitative technique. The gating of small particles continues to be a challenge but flow cytomtery continues to be the only robust technique which can demonstrate the cell of origin for the MP. This is an important asset of flow cytometry. However, there is significant variability amongst flow cytometers and the ISTH subcommittee on vascular biology recently conducted a workshop on standardization of MP by flow cytometry (Lacroix). It remains a popular approach for detection of MP for the following reasons:1)Rapid turn around time 2)Both fresh and frozen specimens may be used 3)The expression of two or more antigens on the MP may be simultaneously demonstrated 4)Easy method for quantification using commercial beads.

However it has the following drawbacks: 1) The detection of particles less than 0.3μm is difficult by flow cytometry as the detection is limited by particle size in the same order of magnitude wavelength of the laser (about 488 nm 2) Different machines have different sensitivities 3) It is difficult to automate 4) Centrifugation speeds for sample processing are variable and not standardized (Freyssinet, 2005). Several new approaches to flow cytometry include using impedance flow cytometry and using Raman microspectrophotometry effect to cover the size and particle discrimination issues (Ayers, 2011).

The capture of MP into immobilized annexin V or cell specific antibodies using an ELISA based assay have ben the other major approaches (Enjeti, 2007). Solid phase assays have the advantage of picking up microparticles irrespective of size. However interference of soluble antigens, variable quality of antibodies used for antigen capture and non-exclusion of microsomes are some of the disadvantages.

4.3 Nanoscale and newer technologies

In the recent years there has been an adaptation of nanoscale technologies such as atomic force microscopy and nanoparticle measurement techniques. These methods claim to accurately measure particles in the nanoscale size range (Yuana). For example , one such nanoscale technique uses the brownian motion of these small particles to detect and measure them (Harrison, 2009). These methods are expensive, intensive to perform and not yet widely available (Lawrie, 2009). Moreover, the clinical utility of such techniques is not yet established. Recently a proteomic approach to analysis of MP has been described, however, the clinical utility of this approach is also as yet unkown (Howes ; Ramacciotti). Automated devices to analyse MP are also being developed (Wagner, 2010).

4.4 Measuring microparticles: Future directions

There are several outstanding issues such as standardization of preanalytical and analytical variables as well as integration of the various approaches in measuring MP. Several novel approaches are now being considered. 'Megamix beads' is novel approach to standardizing of gating of microparticles using flow cytometry. It uses a mix of a 0.9um and 0.3um sized beads to try and capture all events within the gate set by the beads (Robert, 2009 ;Robert, 2011). One of the problems of using this approach is the lack of linearity in the relationship between the size of beads and forward sctatter at that particle size. A recent commercially available nanoscale technology known as 'Nanosight' has incorporated antibody tagging of small particles for accurate identification and counting in this size range (Harrison, 2009).

5. Conclusions

Utility of Measuring MP in venous thromboembolism is yet to be fully established . The case for measuring MP in cancer related VTE is perhaps stronger. There are three areas within which the potential for detecting and measuring MP with respect to venous thromboembolism may be relevant.

5.1 Diagnostic

The evidence for using measurement of MP in a diagnostic setting is limited. The studies so far have shown variable results depending on whether TF bearing MP, functional activity or total MP were measured. With respect to VTE MP have been assessed in the paradigm of VTE, diagnosis in a small pilot study where it was shown that D-dimer, P-selectin and total MP levels predicted thrombosis as demonstrated on Doppler ultrasound (Ramacciotti; Rectenwald, 2005). The role of MP in diagnosis of VTE warrants confirmation in prospective cohort studies. The standardization of measurement of MP will go a long way in ensuring comparability of such studies.

5.2 Prognostic

The potential for MP as a prognostic tool is dependent on reliable, reproducible and easily available tools to measure microparticles. There is emerging data that MP may predict VTE in cancer patients and may be able to provide prognostic information in several other conditions.

5.3 Therapeutic

An interesting dimension to this area is the approach to use or modify MP for therapeutic benefit. The possibility of bioengineered and/or harvested membrane microparticles in tissue repair or angiogenesis is being investigated (Soleti, 2009). The MP are also being studied as a drug delivery tool (Benameur, 2009). Microparticles could potentially be specifically targeted to reduce or prevent thrombotic complications or end organ damage (Myers, 2005). This is an promising and exciting new area for researchers and clinicians working in this area.

Microparticles have therefore emerged as key role players in vascular biology and pathophysiology of thrombosis. They remain an important research tool and their clinical applications are being actively investigated with potential to be applied in diagnostic, prognostic and therapeutic arenas. They are small yet powerful effectors for the pathophysiology of the endovascular system.

6. References

Ahn, Y.S. (2005) Cell-derived microparticles: 'Miniature envoys with many faces'. *J Thromb Haemost,* 3, 884-887.

Ay, C., Freyssinet, J.M., Sailer, T., Vormittag, R. & Pabinger, I. (2009) Circulating procoagulant microparticles in patients with venous thromboembolism. *Thrombosis research,* 123, 724-726.

Biro, E., Sturk-Maquelin, K.N., Vogel, G.M., Meuleman, D.G., Smit, M.J., Hack, C.E., Sturk, A. & Nieuwland, R. (2003) Human cell-derived microparticles promote thrombus formation in vivo in a tissue factor-dependent manner. *J Thromb Haemost,* 1, 2561-2568.

Chirinos, J.A., Heresi, G.A., Velasquez, H., Jy, W., Jimenez, J.J., Ahn, E., Horstman, L.L., Soriano, A.O., Zambrano, J.P. & Ahn, Y.S. (2005) Elevation of endothelial microparticles, platelets, and leukocyte activation in patients with venous thromboembolism. *J Am Coll Cardiol,* 45, 1467-1471.

Collen, D. & Hoylaerts, M.F. (2005) Relationship between inflammation and venous thromboembolism as studied by microparticle assessment in plasma. *Journal of the American College of Cardiology,* 45, 1472-1473.

Combes, V., Simon, A.C., Grau, G.E., Arnoux, D., Camoin, L., Sabatier, F., Mutin, M., Sanmarco, M., Sampol, J. & Dignat-George, F. (1999) In vitro generation of endothelial microparticles and possible prothrombotic activity in patients with lupus anticoagulant. *J Clin Invest,* 104, 93-102.

Diaz, C. & Schroit, A.J. (1996) Role of translocases in the generation of phosphatidylserine asymmetry. *J Membr Biol,* 151, 1-9.

Dignat-George, F., Camoin-Jau, L., Sabatier, F., Arnoux, D., Anfosso, F., Bardin, N., Veit, V., Combes, V., Gentile, S., Moal, V., Sanmarco, M. & Sampol, J. (2004) Endothelial microparticles: a potential contribution to the thrombotic complications of the antiphospholipid syndrome. *Thromb Haemost,* 91, 667-673.

Eilertsen, K.E. & Osterud, B. (2004) Tissue factor: (patho)physiology and cellular biology. *Blood Coagul Fibrinolysis,* 15, 521-538.

Enjeti, A.K., Lincz, L.F., Scorgie, F.E. & Seldon, M. Circulating microparticles are elevated in carriers of factor V Leiden. *Thromb Res,* 126, 250-253.

Enjeti, A.K., Lincz, L.F. & Seldon, M. (2010) Detection and measurement of microparticles: an evolving research tool for vascular biology. *Semin Thromb Hemost,* 33, 771-779.

Enjeti, A.K., Lincz, L.F. & Seldon, M. (2008) Microparticles in health and disease. *Semin Thromb Hemost,* 34, 683-691.

Falati, S., Liu, Q., Gross, P., Merrill-Skoloff, G., Chou, J., Vandendries, E., Celi, A., Croce, K., Furie, B.C. & Furie, B. (2003) Accumulation of tissue factor into developing thrombi in vivo is dependent upon microparticle P-selectin glycoprotein ligand 1 and platelet P-selectin. *J Exp Med,* 197, 1585-1598.

Freyssinet, J.M. (2003) Cellular microparticles: what are they bad or good for? *J Thromb Haemost,* 1, 1655-1662.

Freyssinet, J.M. & Dignat-George, F. (2005) More on: Measuring circulating cell-derived microparticles. *J Thromb Haemost,* 3, 613-614.

Furie, B. & Furie, B.C. (2004) Role of platelet P-selectin and microparticle PSGL-1 in thrombus formation. *Trends Mol Med,* 10, 171-178.

Furie, B. & Furie, B.C. (2006) Cancer-associated thrombosis. *Blood Cells Mol Dis,* 36, 177-181.

Garcia Rodriguez, P., Eikenboom, H.C., Tesselaar, M.E., Huisman, M.V., Nijkeuter, M., Osanto, S. & Bertina, R.M. (2010) Plasma levels of microparticle-associated tissue factor activity in patients with clinically suspected pulmonary embolism. *Thrombosis research,* 126, 345-349.

Gyorgy, B., Modos, K., Pallinger, E., Paloczi, K., Pasztoi, M., Misjak, P., Deli, M.A., Sipos, A., Szalai, A., Voszka, I., Polgar, A., Toth, K., Csete, M., Nagy, G., Gay, S., Falus, A., Kittel, A. & Buzas, E.I. Detection and isolation of cell-derived microparticles are compromised by protein complexes resulting from shared biophysical parameters. *Blood,* 117, e39-48.

Horstman, L.L., Jy, W., Jimenez, J.J., Bidot, C. & Ahn, Y.S. (2004) New horizons in the analysis of circulating cell-derived microparticles. *Keio J Med,* 53, 210-230.

Horstman, L.L., Jy, W., Minagar, A., Bidot, C.J., Jimenez, J.J., Alexander, J.S. & Ahn, Y.S. (2007) Cell-derived microparticles and exosomes in neuroinflammatory disorders. *Int Rev Neurobiol,* 79, 227-268.

Jy, W., Horstman, L.L. & Ahn, Y.S. Microparticle size and its relation to composition, functional activity, and clinical significance. *Semin Thromb Hemost,* 36, 876-880.

Jy, W., Jimenez, J.J., Mauro, L.M., Horstman, L.L., Cheng, P., Ahn, E.R., Bidot, C.J. & Ahn, Y.S. (2005) Endothelial microparticles induce formation of platelet aggregates via a von Willebrand factor/ristocetin dependent pathway, rendering them resistant to dissociation. *J Thromb Haemost,* 3, 1301-1308.

Jy, W., Tiede, M., Bidot, C.J., Horstman, L.L., Jimenez, J.J., Chirinos, J. & Ahn, Y.S. (2007) Platelet activation rather than endothelial injury identifies risk of thrombosis in subjects positive for antiphospholipid antibodies. *Thromb Res.*

Key, N.S. Analysis of tissue factor positive microparticles. *Thromb Res,* 125 Suppl 1, S42-45.

Key, N.S. & Kwaan, H.C. Microparticles in thrombosis and hemostasis. *Semin Thromb Hemost,* 36, 805-806.

Lawrie, A.S., Albanyan, A., Cardigan, R.A., Mackie, I.J. & Harrison, P. (2009) Microparticle sizing by dynamic light scattering in fresh-frozen plasma. *Vox Sang,* 96, 206-212.

Lozito, T.P. & Tuan, R.S. Endothelial cell microparticles act as centers of Matrix Metalloproteinsase-2 (MMP-2) activation and vascular matrix remodeling. *J Cell Physiol.*

Mallat, Z., Benamer, H., Hugel, B., Benessiano, J., Steg, P.G., Freyssinet, J.M. & Tedgui, A. (2000) Elevated levels of shed membrane microparticles with procoagulant potential in the peripheral circulating blood of patients with acute coronary syndromes. *Circulation,* 101, 841-843.

Mause, S.F., Weber, C., Sampol, J. & Dignat-George, F. New horizons in vascular biology and thrombosis: Highlights from EMVBM 2009. *Thromb Haemost,* 104, 421-423.

Meziani, F., Delabranche, X., Asfar, P. & Toti, F. Bench-to-bedside review: circulating microparticles--a new player in sepsis? *Crit Care,* 14, 236.

Montoro-Garcia, S., Shantsila, E., Marin, F., Blann, A. & Lip, G.Y. Circulating microparticles: new insights into the biochemical basis of microparticle release and activity. *Basic Res Cardiol.*

Morel, O., Jesel, L., Freyssinet, J.M. & Toti, F. Cellular mechanisms underlying the formation of circulating microparticles. *Arterioscler Thromb Vasc Biol,* 31, 15-26.

Morel, O., Toti, F., Hugel, B., Bakouboula, B., Camoin-Jau, L., Dignat-George, F. & Freyssinet, J.M. (2006) Procoagulant microparticles: disrupting the vascular homeostasis equation? *Arterioscler Thromb Vasc Biol,* 26, 2594-2604.

Owen, B.A., Xue, A., Heit, J.A. & Owen, W.G. Procoagulant activity, but not number, of microparticles increases with age and in individuals after a single venous thromboembolism. *Thromb Res,* 127, 39-46.

Pilzer, D., Gasser, O., Moskovich, O., Schifferli, J.A. & Fishelson, Z. (2005) Emission of membrane vesicles: roles in complement resistance, immunity and cancer. *Springer Semin Immunopathol,* 27, 375-387.

Porto, I., De Maria, G.L., Di Vito, L., Camaioni, C., Gustapane, M. & Biasucci, L.M. Microparticles in Health and Disease: Small Mediators, Large Role? *Curr Vasc Pharmacol.*

Rectenwald, J.E., Myers, D.D., Jr., Hawley, A.E., Longo, C., Henke, P.K., Guire, K.E., Schmaier, A.H. & Wakefield, T.W. (2005) D-dimer, P-selectin, and microparticles: novel markers to predict deep venous thrombosis. A pilot study. *Thromb Haemost,* 94, 1312-1317.

Shantsila, E., Kamphuisen, P.W. & Lip, G.Y. Circulating microparticles in cardiovascular disease: implications for atherogenesis and atherothrombosis. *J Thromb Haemost,* 8, 2358-2368.

Siljander, P., Carpen, O. & Lassila, R. (1996) Platelet-derived microparticles associate with fibrin during thrombosis. *Blood,* 87, 4651-4663.

Siljander, P.R. Platelet-derived microparticles - an updated perspective. *Thromb Res,* 127 Suppl 2, S30-33.

Simak, J. & Gelderman, M.P. (2006) Cell membrane microparticles in blood and blood products: potentially pathogenic agents and diagnostic markers. *Transfus Med Rev,* 20, 1-26.

Soleti, R., Benameur, T., Porro, C., Panaro, M.A., Andriantsitohaina, R. & Martinez, M.C. (2009) Microparticles harboring Sonic Hedgehog promote angiogenesis through the upregulation of adhesion proteins and proangiogenic factors. *Carcinogenesis,* 30, 580-588.

Soleti, R. & Martinez, M.C. (2009) Microparticles harbouring Sonic Hedgehog: role in angiogenesis regulation. *Cell adhesion & migration,* 3, 293-295.

SSCMembers (Aug 2005) Working group on vascular biology. Minutes of the SSC organizing committee. *ISTH annual meeting Sydney.*

Thaler, J., Ay, C., Weinstabl, H., Dunkler, D., Simanek, R., Vormittag, R., Freyssinet, J.M., Zielinski, C. & Pabinger, I. Circulating procoagulant microparticles in cancer patients. *Ann Hematol,* 90, 447-453.

Walenga, J.M., Jeske, W.P. & Messmore, H.L. (2000) Mechanisms of venous and arterial thrombosis in heparin-induced thrombocytopenia. *J Thromb Thrombolysis,* 10 Suppl 1, 13-20.

Yuana, Y., Oosterkamp, T.H., Bahatyrova, S., Ashcroft, B., Garcia Rodriguez, P., Bertina, R.M. & Osanto, S. Atomic force microscopy: a novel approach to the detection of nanosized blood microparticles. *J Thromb Haemost,* 8, 315-323.

Zwaal, R.F., Comfurius, P. & Bevers, E.M. (2004) Scott syndrome, a bleeding disorder caused by defective scrambling of membrane phospholipids. *Biochim Biophys Acta,* 1636, 119-128.

Zwaal, R.F., Comfurius, P. & Bevers, E.M. (2005) Surface exposure of phosphatidylserine in pathological cells. *Cell Mol Life Sci,* 62, 971-988.

2

Hyperhomocysteinemia: Relation to Cardiovascular Disease and Venous Thromboembolism

Nadja Plazar and Mihaela Jurdana
University of Primorska, College of Health Care Izola, Slovenia

1. Introduction

Homocysteine is a sulphur-containing amino acid, which structurally is closely related to the essential amino acids methionine and cysteine. The cellular methylation cycle performs the metabolism of methionine and since homocysteine is an intermediate within this cycle, the body in this way is provided with all organic homocysteine. The term homocysteine is used to define the combined pool of homocysteine, homocystine, and mixed disulfide compounds (Fig. 1) even involving homocysteine thiolactone a cyclic form which is often found in the plasma of patients with hyperhomocisteinemia.

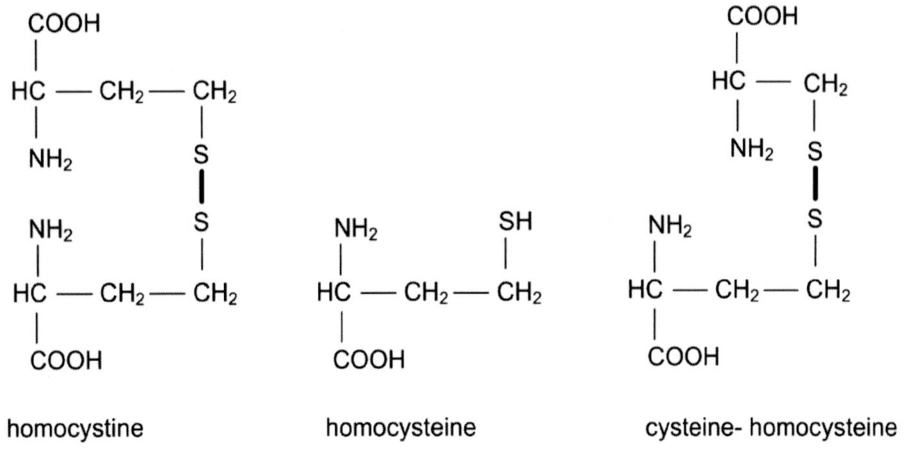

Fig. 1. Structural formulae of homocysteine

Homocysteine was first isolated by Butz and du Vigneaud in 1932. However, the relation of homocysteine to human disease was first suggested in 1962, in the classical paper of Carson and Neil, reporting an elevated homocysteine level in the urine of mentally retarded children. Nowadays, it has long been known that homocystinuria—also known as severe hyperhomocysteinemia, a genetic disorder in which blood levels of homocysteine are about 20-fold higher than the normal concentration—is associated with greatly increased risk for premature vascular disease, occlusive cardiovascular disease in early life and childhood, leading to incidental strokes or heart attacks in teenagers. It is caused by inherited metabolic defects of the homocysteine metabolism, and is therefore positively correlated with a very high risk of venous thromboembolism (VTE), (Mudd et al., 1970).

These observations raised the question whether moderately elevated plasma homocysteine concentrations, often called moderate hyperhomocisteinemia, may also cause irritation of the blood vessels and are a risk factor for cardiovascular disesase (CVD) in general (McCully, 1960). McCully proposed that elevated homocysteine can cause atherosclerotic vascular disease (McCully, 1960). Early support for this concept came from a study published in 1976 by Wilcken and Wilcken, who reported that, following an oral dose of methionine, serum homocysteine levels tended to be higher in patients with premature coronary disease than in healthy controls (Wilcken & Wilcken, 1976).

Mild or moderate hyperhomocysteinemia which occurs in the health population with a frequency of 5 to 7 % is often caused by the interaction of environmental factors with mild genetic abnormalities of homocysteine metabolism.

Venous thrombosis was clearly described in patients with mild/moderate homocysteinuria and since then, several case-control and prospective studies showed the association with increased risk of VTE, (Mudd et al., 1985). Besides, also a large number of retrospective studies show that mildly elevated homocysteine levels (mild/moderate hyperhomocysteinemia caused by the interaction of envirovmental factors with mild genetic abnormalities of homocysteine metabolism) are associated with VTE. Only recently, an elevated homocysteine level has also been established as a risk factor for venous thrombosis (Moll, 2004). Moreover, in patients with venous thrombosis elevated homocysteine levels have attracted considerable interest because homocysteine is an easy to monitor thrombophilic marker, and thus can indicate the time and need for measures, to potentially reverse the venous thrombosis (Cattaneo, 2006).

Because of the already high prevalence of (hyper/moderate/mild) homocysteinemia in the healthly population and people with disease, this review focusses the attention on (1) the relevance of the metabolic pathway of homocysteine, (2) the importance of dietary intake of folate, vitamines B6 and B12 and (3) the recommendations to modify life style factors in order to prevent, in general, a further homocysteinemia-induced increase of the VTE and cardiovascular disease complications.

2. Homocysteine metabolism

2.1 Plasma homocysteine

As mentioned in the introduction homocysteine is a sulfur-containing intermediate in the normal metabolism of the essential amino acid methionine, occuring in almost all body cells and in general 5 to 10% of the daily synthesized homocysteine (1.2 mmol/day) is transferred into the blood through hepatocytes (Weisberg et al., 2003). Besides, proliferating cells secrete more homocysteine compared to non-proliferating cells. Although plasma concentrations of homocysteine vary widely, on the other hand the intracellular concentrations are preserved within a narrow range (Moat et al., 2004). In the plasma, about circa 90% homocysteine is protein-bound, while circa 10% is present as the cysteine mixed disulphide and less than 1% is present in the free reduced form. The total plasma level includes the summed amount of all the homocysteine forms in the circulation (Hankey & Eikelboom, 1999).

Normal and abnormal homocysteine levels are set by individual laboratories. Typically, considered normal is less than 13 µmol/L, between 13 and 60 µmol/L is considered moderately elevated, and higher than 60 to 100 µmol/L is severely elevated (Moll, 2004). The total plasma homocysteine concentrations during hyperhomocysteinemia are between 12 and 30 µmol/L, with gender differences being present. Higher values are measured in men, and apparently the presence of estrogen in women determines the plasma concentration after the menopause the blood levels of homocysteine of woman approximate those in men (Ridker et al., 1999), Table1.

Sex	Age	Lower limit	Upper limit	Unit	Moderatelly elevated
Female	12-19 years	3.3	7.2	µmol/L	13-60 µmol/L
	>60 years	5	12	µmol/L	
Male	12-19 years	4.3	9.9	µmol/L	> 11.4 µmol/L
	>60 years	6	15.3	µmol/L	

Table 1. Blood reference ranges for homocysteine

The homocysteine levels are measured through a routine blood test, where blood samples are collected in EDTA or citrate anticoagulant tubes and should be centrifuged and the plasma separated immediately. Ideally, the homocysteine is measured in overnight fasting subjects, since high-protein meals will influence the results. Another test, the methionine-load test measures the homocysteine levels before and after the intake of 100 mg/kg of methionine and can be used to diagnose abnormal homocysteine metabolism in people with a high risk for cardiovascular disesase, but who have normal homocysteine concentration during fasting. This test can be used to make decisions about therapy.

Homocysteine exists in plasma in a free and a bound form. The determination measures the total homocysteine level is the sum of all forms. The commercial methods of determination include the transformation of all forms of homocysteine, by means or reduction, into total homocysteine, which than is quantified by different methods: gas chromatography, mass spectrometry, high pressure liquid chromatography and the most frequently commercial methods as florescence polarization immunoassay, chemiluminescence immunoassay, or enzyme-linked immunoassay, used on different analyzers.

Results obtained with different methods are often not very com-parable each other because of considerable inter-method and inter-laboratory variability. Reported approaches for the measurement of plasma tHcys include: ion-exchange chromatography, immunoassays (fluorescence polarization immunoassay, FPIA, or chemiluminescence immunoassay, ICL,or enzyme-linked immunoassay, EIA), HPLC (with photometric, fluorescence or electrochemical detection),capillary electrophoresis with photometricor laser fluorescence detec- tion), GC–MS,and LC–ESI-MS/MS. Many of them have significant disadvantages, including derivatization protocols, are expensive and time-consuming. Compared with the above mentioned, LC–ESI-MS/MS seems to be the most suitable method because of its inherent accuracy, high sensitivity, specificity and high through put for t Hcys analysis.

2.2 Role of B vitamins and enzymes

B vitamins function as coenzymes in the synthesis of purines and thymidylate during normal DNA synthesis. Diminished levels of these vitamins may result in misincorporation of uracil into DNA, leading to chromosome breaks and disruption of DNA repair and both, folate and vitamin B12 levels are involved in DNA methylation. Deficient folate and vitamin B12 levels can reduce the availability of S-adenosylmethionine, the universal methyl donor, for DNA methylation and may thereby influence gene expression (Blount et al., 1997).

Some people have elevated homocysteine levels due to an unbalanced diet with suboptimal intake of B vitamins (B6, B12 and folate), which act as coenzymes in the metabolism of homocysteine (de Bree et al., 1997, Stanger et al., 2003). Several studies have found that high blood levels of B vitamins influence the integrity and function of DNA, and, correlate with a low concentration of homocysteine, while folate depletion has been found to change DNA methylation and DNA synthesis in both animal and human studies.

B vitamines are very important in the transformation of homocysteine in methionine and are cofactors to three important enzymes directly involved in the homocysteine metabolism: (1) methionine synthase (MS), (2) methylenetetrahydrofolatereductase (MTHFR) and (3) cystathione β-synthase (CBS).

Therefore, deficiencies of folate and vitamin B12 and reduced activity of the involved metabolic enzymes will inhibit the breakdown of homocysteine, leading to an accumulation of the intracellular homocysteine, followed by rapid excretion to the circulation and eventually increased plasma levels (Silaste et al., 2001).

Via the trans-sulfuration pathway homocysteine is converted into cystathionine to form cysteine by cystathionine-ß-synthase, with vitamin B6 as a co-factor. Another pathway of homocysteine metabolism is the re-methylation pathway, which is connected with the folate metabolic pathway (Fig. 2). It involves the transfer of a methyl group from 5-methyl-tetrahydrofolate to homocysteine to form methionine, and eventually S-adenosylmethionine. The methyl transfer from 5-methyl tetrahydrofolate to homocysteine is catalyzed by methionine-synthase, and requires vitamin B12 as a cofactor. Important to notice is that S-adenosylmethionine is the universal methyl donor for methylation reactions. The resulting tetrahydrofolate transfers into the 5,10-methyltetrahydrofolate with the enzyme 5,10-methyltetrahydrofolate reductase (MTHFR) and then into the 5-methyltetrahydrofolate 5-MTHF, (Fodinger et al., 2000). The cellular availability of 5-MTHF may be of great importance in regulating cellular effects of homocysteine related to cell growth.

The methyl group of 5-MTHF is transported to vitamin B12 linked to the enzyme homocysteine-methyl-transferase to yield methylcobalamin-enzyme. This complex adds the methyl group to homocysteine to form methionine (Pietrzik & Brönstrup, 1998).

Therefore, deficiencies of folate and vitamin B12 and reduced activity of the involved metabolic enzymes will inhibit the breakdown of homocysteine, which will lead to an increase of the intracellular homocysteine concentration (Silaste et al., 2001).

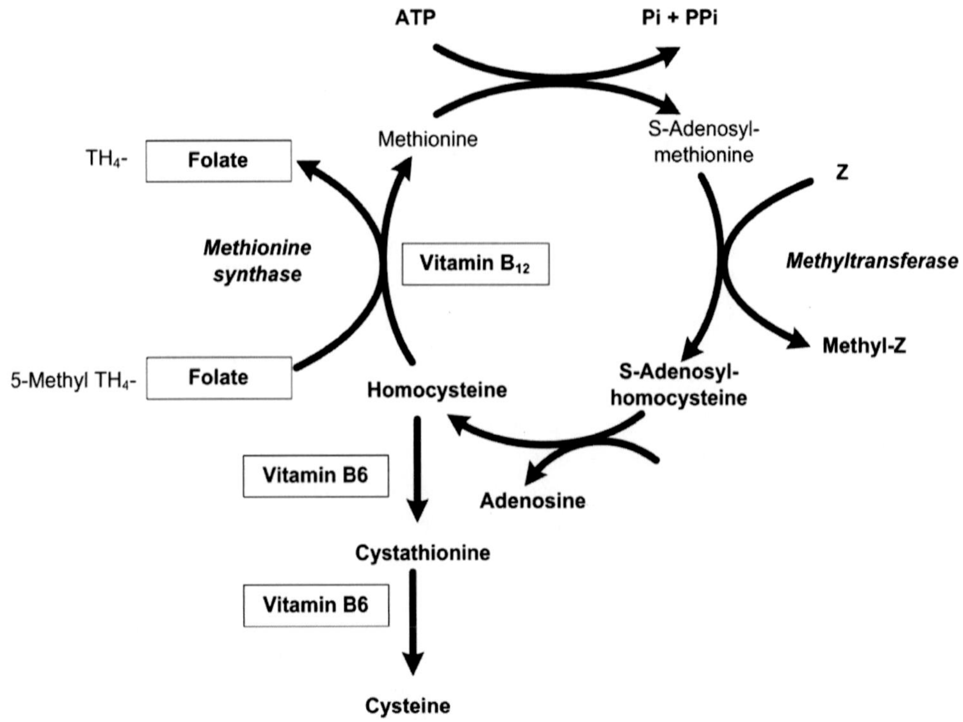

Fig. 2. Homocysteine metabolism

S-adenosylhomocysteine is formed during S-adenosylmethionine-dependent methylation reactions, and the hydrolysis of S-adenosylhomocysteine results in homocysteine. Homocysteine may be remethylated to form methionine by a folate-dependent reaction that is catalyzed by methionine synthase, a vitamin B12-dependent enzyme. Alternately, homocysteine may be metabolized to cysteine in reactions catalyzed by two vitamin B6-dependent enzymes.

3. Causes of hyperhomocysteinemia

3.1 Genetic deffects

Elevation in plasma homocysteine are typically caused either by genetic defects in the enzymes involved in homocysteine metabolism or by nutritional deficiencies in vitamin cofactors. Homocysteinuria and severe hyperhomocystenemia are caused by rare inborn errors of metabolism resulting in marked elevations of plasma and urine homocysteine concentrations.

Most studies refer to changes in the cystathionine β-synthase gene or in the GCT gene (γ cystathionase), both coding the trans-sulfuration pathway (references). Further, mutations do occur in the genes coding for the enzymes involved. Cystathionine β-synthase (CBS) deficiency is the most common genetic cause of severe hyperhomocysteinemia. As first shown in a study by Carey and colleagues as early as 1968, the homozygous form of this disease – congenital homocystinuria – can be associated with hyperhomocysteinemia, and in these homozygotes there is a frequent development of atherothrombotic complications during young adulthood, which often are fatal. Mudd and colleagues estimated that approximately 50 percent of untreated homocystinuria patients will have a thromboembolic event before the age of 30 and that the disease-related mortality is approximately 20 percent (Mudd et al., 1970).

Other abnormalities of the remethylation cycle that are associated with hyperhomocysteinemia include genetic methionine synthase deficiency and genetic disorders of vitamin B_{12} metabolism both impairing methionine synthase activity.

Genetic mutations in MTHFR are the most commonly known inherited risk factor for elevated homocysteine levels. To have any detrimental effect, mutations must be present in both copies of a person's MTHFR genes (Varga et al., 2005). (1) A point mutation in the coding region for the 5,10-MTHFR binding site (C677T), leading to the substitution of an alanine to a valine effectively increases homocysteine levels increase and decreases methionine levels or (2) A1298C another common point mutation of the MTHFR gene, both affect the enzyme activity catalyzing the vitamin B_{12}-dependent remethylation of homocysteine to methionine. C677T homozygotes carry the double TT (thermolabile) allele of the enzyme MTHFR gene of which the enzyme activity is reduced to 35% of the normal (Schriver et al., 1995), and having an average homocysteine level of 19.7 μM. In CT heterocygotes this is 10.3 μM, while for CC unaffected this is 10.0 μM. Further, data show that people with C677T TT have 21% increased risk of ischemic heart disease; in those with CT the risk is increased by only 6% (Dinesh -K, 2004).

Aproximally 10% to 20% of Caucasians carry the TT allele, whereas the remaining 80% - 90% carry either the CT or CC alleles. Black subjects have a very low frequency of carring the TT allele. The C677T mutation does have different regional incidences in Europe where the German and Italian populations show different incidences of 24.5% and 43.8% respectively.

3.2 Other disease states

Hyperhomocysteinemia occurrs in a wide range of unrelated diseases as depicted in Table 1.

Over the past 15 years, there has been an explosion in the number of scientific articles describing an association between homocysteine and vascular disease. Hyperhomocysteinemia has been linked to an increased risk of cardiac events; sudden death; stroke; coronary- carotid- cerebral- and peripheral-arterial diseases. It is also implicated in transplant coronary artery disease and essential hypertension (Dinesh, 2004). In general, retrospective analyses show that for every 4 μM rise in homocysteine levels, the relative risk for cardio vascular disease increases by 1.3 to 1.4 (Nygard et al. 1997a). Data obtained from (COMAC-European concerted Action Project (Graham et al., 1997), which studied patients with vascular disease and control subjects, confirmed that homocysteine levels more than 12 μM increased the risk for all types of atherotrombotic vascular disease. So, after a thorough review of the available literature, hyperhomocysteinemia should be considered an independent risk factor for cardiovascular disease.

Aging	Heart conditions
Alzheimers disease	Mental retardation
Anaemias	Migraines
Angina	Miscarriages
Arthritis	Osteoporosis
Artheriosclerosis	Parkinson's disease
Auto-immune diseases	Polycystic ovary disease
Birth defects	Pregnancy complications
Cancers	Psoriasis
Cholesterol - high	Rheumatoid arthritis
Chronic fatigue	Schizophrenia
Coeliac disease	Strokes
Chrohn's disease	Thyroid disorders
Depression	Ulcerative colitis
Diabetes	Epilepsy

Table 2. Common diseases associated with high homocysteine levels (Hultberg et al., 1993; Pettersson et al., 1998; Bolander-Gouaille, 2001; Hultberg, 1993).

3.3 Lifestyle factors

From a public health viewpoint, it is important to identify modifiable factors that influence the plasma homocysteine concentrations. The next lifestyle factors may have an effect on plasma homocysteine concentration (Bolander-Gouaille, 2001):

3.3.1 Smoking

Smoking is associated with vascular disease and other complications related to homocysteine (Bolander-Gouaille, 2001). The number of cigarettes smoked a day was one of the strongest determinants of homocysteine levels (Nygard et al., 1995). In women, the increase of plasma homocysteine levels was about 1% per each cigarette smoked, and in men about 0.5%. The mechanisms by which smoking increases the homocysteine levels may be manifold, however there is some experimental evidence that nicotine directly affects the methylation reactions. Besides, in smokers catabolism of folate has been suggested(Godin & Crooks, 1986).

3.3.2 High alcohol intake

High alcohol consumption is often associated with gastrointestinal disturbances, which may result in decrease absorption of vitamins (the most important is folic acid), thus contributing to elevated homocysteine levels. Alcohol has also been reported to inhibit methionine synthase (MS), to decrease hepatic uptake and increase excretion, mainly via urine (Barak et al., 1993). The decreased concentration of serum folic acid may occur in 80% of alcohol abusers and this can lead to serious clinical consequences.

3.3.3 Coffee consumption

Coffee consumption has been associated with several risk factors for coronary heart disease, including plasma total homocysteine and reduced B vitamin concentrations (Ulvike et al., 2008). Coffee drinking is associated with smoking and low intake of fruit and vegetables. Tea consumption, in contrast, was associated with lower homocysteine levels (Nygard et al., 1997b).

3.3.4 Inadequate nutrition

B vitamins have been suggested to play a critical role to maintain low homocysteine levels (Silaste et al., 2001). A diet poor in fresh fruit and vegetables or strict vegeterians may develop nutritional vitamin B12 deficiency (Miller et al., 1991). This is particulary serious in pregnancy, as the mother may not be able to supply the fetus with sufficient vitamin B12. Also modern food processing may destroy essential vitamins and it has recently been shown that microwave heating may destroy as much as 30 % of the vitamin B12 content in food (Watanabe et al., 1998). Prolonged heating may also destroy folate and vitamin B6. Besides, healthly subjects eating fish more than 3 times a week had lower homocysteine levels than those eating fish less than one a month.

3.3.5 Physical activity

Physical activity plays an important role in our life, since it is the cheapest way of strengthening our health and reduces the risk of developing cardiovascular diseases. It has been confirmed that physical activity decreases the concentrations of total plasma homocysteine and thus the probability of developing a cardiovascular disease in healthy and already sick people. In the study called Bed rest "The influence of simulated weightlessness upon the human organism" performed in 2006, 2007 and 2008 at the Valdoltra Orthopaedic Hospital, Slovenia, in which young male participants (age 24-30 years) rested in horizontal position for 35 days, a statistically increased homocysteine concentration was documented (Plazar et al., 2008). The diet composition and the energy intake were daily supervised and monitored by a dietician. Volunteers were non-smokers, non-alcoholics, without history of cardiovascular and neuromuscular disorders. Several studies indicate physical activity as an independent lifestyle factor connected with lower homocysteine concentration. Besides, exercise is associated with a reduction in plasma fibrinogen concentrations, and with increasing activity levels of exercise a reduction in homocysteine was observed. So, this prolonged bed rest study confirms that increased levels of homocysteine in blood, negatively influences the cardiovascular system. Although, the precise mechanism is not well understood, similar consequences can result from prolonged physical inactivity in everyday life.

3.3.6 Age related factors

Many studies have shown that hyperhomocysteinemia increases with age (Pennypacker et al., 1992). This is connected with inadequate nutrition, the changes in gastrointestinal function, B vitamins deficiency, enzyme defects, a higher occurance of the C677T mutation and numerous age-related physiological factors.

MOST COMMON RISK FACTORS
Inherited
CBS deficiency
MTHFR deficiency
MS deficiency
Being male
Aquired
Aged 40 +
Deficients of folate, vitamin B6 and B12
Post menopausal status
Drinking alcohol
Smoking
Often angry or suppress anger
Physical inactivity / sedentary life-style
Drinking caffeinated drinks - coffee, tea, coke
Being pregnant
Being strict vegetarian
High fat/protein diet intake
High diet salt intake
Hypothyroidism
Chronic kidney problems
Use drugs: e.g.: phenytoin, carbamazepine, methotrexate, aminoglutethimide
Suffering from chronic illnesses
Digestive problems, auto-immune diseases, asthma, eczema, arthritis, osteoporosis, ulcers, diabetes, heart conditions, high blood pressure, thrombosis, cancer

Table 3. Common risk factors inducing mild hyperhomocysteinemia

4. Venous thromoembolism and hyperhomocysteinemia

It has been recognized, since the first description of hyperhomocysteinemia, that arterial and venous thrombosis are common in these patients. Patients with homocysteinuria suffered of thrombotic events, cerebrovascular occlusions, deep vein thromboses, myocardial infarctions and peripheral vascular thromboses (Mudd et al., 1985) of which a quarter of all thrombotic events occured before the age of 16 and half before the age of 28, much earlier in life than would normally be expected for these types of events. Further, patients with CBS deficiency-induced homocysteinuria have high levels of plasma homocysteine (Carey et al., 1968). Interest in the hyperhomocysteinemia condition increased when a large number of studies (mainly retrospective) showed that also mildly elevated homocysteine levels are associated with venous thromboembolism (VTE), thrombotic stroke, and peripheral vascular disease (Wilcken & Wilcken, 1976, Mudd et al., 1985, Moll, 2004).

To conclude, mild hyperhomocysteinemia can be induced by a variety of risk factors of which the most common genetic factors are heterozygous CBS gene defects and polymorphism in the MTHFR gene at position 677, while as well numerous aquired conditions might be involved (Table 3).

Independent from other factors hyperhomocysteinemia is associated with a 4.8 fold increased risk for VTE (Köktürk et al., 2010).

4.1 Mechanisms for thrombosis in hyperhomocysteinemia

Homocysteine impairs intrinsic thrombolysis and endothelium function (Dalton et al., 1997; Nishio & Watanabe; 1997). Studies of cultured cells in vitro indicate that homocysteine has prothrombotic effects on the endothelium and vascular smooth muscle. *In vitro* test results show that endothelial cells are damaged by moderate hyperhomocysteinemia mainly because of the impact of hydrogen peroxide (Hultberg et al., 1997).

Homocysteine though oxidative stress, probably directly damages endothelial cells by: (1) the direct oxidation of low density lipoproteins (2) its cytoplasmic oxidation products like homocystine, mixed disulfides and homocysteine thiolactone, which lead to the development of reactive oxidative species ROS such as hydrogen peroxide, superoxide anion and hydroxide radical (3) acceleration of fibrin and collagen accumulation in endothelial cells and smooth muscle cells, stimulating their proliferation and thus changes the vessel wall leading to or at least accelerating thrombus and vascular disease.

The metabolism of homocysteine is connected with the cellular level of S-adenosyl methionine (SAM) which is a co-substrate involved in methyl group transfers of both the transsulfuration and remethylation metabolic pathways (Fig.2) by the enzyme methyltransferase. At the same time, SAM is the methyl group donor in the methylation of DNA, proteins, phospholipids and biogenic amines. Therefore, the methyltransferase function depends on the cell concentration of both SAM and S-adenosyl homocysteine (SAH). Effectively, high cellular homocysteine levels inhibit vital methylation reactions, affecting the maintenance of the DNA structure; without repair mutations can occur and the structure can collapse. The close connection of homocysteine metabolism with methyl transfer reactions imply, that changed methyl transfer reactions are responsible for some of the effects of altered vessel function during hyperhomocysteinemia.

It is very likely that the mechanisms by which homocysteine changes vessel function are oxidative stress and alterations of cell methylation (Lentz, 1998). The proposed pathogenetic mechanisms which associate hyperhomocysteinemia and vascular injury are oxidative damage of the endothelium through suppression of the vasodilator nitric oxide, increasing the level of asymmetric dimethylarginine, impairing methylation, proliferation of vascular smooth muscle, and disruption of the normal procoagulant balance in favor of thrombosis.

4.2 Homocysteine and thrombosis in malignancies, renal failure, retina veins

4.2.1 Malignancies and VTE

More recently, increased plasma homocysteine concentration has been postulated as a risk factor for cancer and even as a novel tumor marker (Sun et al., 2002). Patients with malignancies often have an increased risk of VTE disease and as such being the second most common cause of death in cancer patients, second to the primary disease itself (Rickles et al., 1992). In 1865 Trousseau described hypercoagulability and increasing risk of »spontaneous coagulation« in patients with cancer (Trousseau, 1865). Nowadays, it is established that breast, pancreas, and gastrointestinal cancers are associated with a higher incidence of thrombosis. With more advanced stages of cancer there is a lower overall survival rate, but, also a greater risk of venous thromboembolism, additionally influencing the survival of patients.

The associated pathophysiology of VTE and malignancies has not been precisely defined. However, it has been reported that cancer patients show increased levels of several pro-coagulant factors (Falanga et al., 1993). It is well established that women with advanced breast cancer show hyperhomocysteinemia, which explains the hight rate of venous thrombosis in women with metastatic breast malignancy (Smith et al., 2008). Other established contributors to the VTE increased risk are: chemotherapy, hormonal adjuvant therapy, surgery, central venous catheters, immobility and inherited thrombophilia, with the notion that oncological therapies do influence the immunological response.

4.2.2 Renal failure and VTE

Under physiological conditions, non-protein bound homocysteine is subjected to glomerular filtration, and almost completely reabsorbed in the tubuli and oxidatively catabolized to carbon dioxide and sulphate in the kidney cells. The clearance is markedly reduced in renal failure with a strong, positive correlation between homocysteine levels, serum creatinine and the glomerular filtration rate (Hultberg et al., 1993). Hyperhomocysteinemia in patients with chronic renal failure induces an oxidative stress to the vascular endothelium, causing a failure in vasodilatation and an impairment of antithrombotic properties. In patients with end-stage renal disease (ESRD) the prevalence of hyperhomocysteinemia is 85-100% and of the fifty-nine ESRD patients undergoing hemodialysis treatment with supplemented B vitamines it was concluded that the MTHFR C677T mutation is an important genetic determinant of elevated plasma homocysteine concentration level.

4.2.3 Retinal Vein occlusion

Several studies have examined the relationship between hyperhomocysteinemia and retinal vein occlusion, a condition affecting approximately five out of 1000 of the general population over 64 years of age (David et al., 1988). The association between retinal vein occlusion, hyperhomocysteinemia and thermolabile MTHFR was confirmed (Janssen et al., 2005).

4.2.4 Homocysteine and thrombosis in children

Venous thrombosis in children occurs at a much lower frequency than in adults and the events are usually provoked by acquired risk factors like sepsis, cancer and central venous catheters. The association of VTE and hyperhomocysteinemia in children has been confirmed in two case control studies (Koch et al., 1999; Kosch et al., 2004).

4.2.5 Hyperhomocysteinemia and pregnancy

Hyperhomocysteinemia during pregnancy, which is a consequence of perturbations in methionine and/or the folate metabolism, has been implicated in adverse outcomes such as neural tube defects, preeclampsia, spontaneous abortion, and premature delivery (Dasarathy et al., 2010). This is pertinent as it is believed that placental thrombosis may contribute to the pathogenesis of these conditions (Gatt & Makris, 2007).

5. Treatment of hyperhomocysteinemia

The treatment of hyperhomocysteinemia varies with the underlying cause.

In the case of deficiency of one or more vitamins involved in homocysteine metabolism, blood levels of this amino acid are often elevated well above those observed in the healthy population. Treatment of hyperhomocysteinemia includes supplementation with mostly pharmacological doses of one or more of the relevant B vitamins and is generally effective in reducing homocysteine concentrations and delays atherosclerotic and thrombotic events.

The negative impact of particular genotypes on homocysteine levels can partly be compensated by folate intake and is, even in smaller part, dependent on several other variables that affect homocysteine levels (see Table 2). For example, if persons have balanced diet with optimal intake of B6 and B12 vitamins and folates it seems that the C677T mutation and the subsequent reduced activity of the enzyme MTHFR do not connect with hyperhomocysteinemia (Schriver et al., 1995; Silaste et al., 2001). Besides, folic acid supplemetation reduces the plasma homocysteine concentration in all three genotypes (TT, CT and CC) of the MTHFR C677T mutation (Meshkin & Blum, 2007).

This scientific evidence suggests that the MTHFR C677T genetic mutation influences folate metabolism, leading to the conclusion that dietary intake of a standard dosage of folate may be insufficient for half to two-thirds of the population with this mutation (Meshkin & Blum, 2007).

In the case of CBS deficiency, the enzyme activity can effectively be enhanced by treatment with large doses of vitamin B6.

A combination of all three relevant coenzymes to treat milder forms of hyperhomocysteinemia resulted in a clear 50% reduction of plasma homocysteine levels. However, given alone, only folic acid was able to induce similar reductions, whereas vitamin B 12 was little effective and vitamin B6 failed to show an effect (Perry et al., 1968, Ubbink et al., 1993; Ubbink et al., 1994).

Many countries have implemented mandatory folic acid fortification of flour and grain products to reduce the risk of various diseases. Besides, individuals can find a good source of folate in fruits and vegetables (especially green leafy vegetables).

6. Who should be tested for MTHFR mutations and homocysteine levels

For individuals with unexplained arterial or venous blood clots and unexplained atherosclerosis it seems appropiate having blood homocysteine levels checked. One can also argue that everybody with atherosclerosis, patients with CVD, heart attacks, or strokes, should have their blood checked for homocysteine levels. All this in order to prevent further damage. At this time, no clear medical indication exists for women with a history of recurrent pregnancy loss, preeclampsia, placental abruption, and/or small-for-age babies to have homocysteine levels checked, although appropiate clinical research should come with more evidence for this.

As with homocysteine, no official guidelines exist as to who should be tested for MTHFR. In the absence of elevated homocysteine levels, MTHFR mutations appear to have no clinical relevance in regard to thrombosis and atherosclerosis. However, in case of elevated homocysteine levels of MTHFR patients the risk for venous thromoembolism increases dramatically. Since treatment can be relatively easy according to diet, one could argue that there is indication to perform MTHFR genetic testing after the homocysteine test shows elevated levels (Varga et al., 2005).

7. Conclusion

Elevated homocysteine concentration has been identified as an independent risk factor for premature cardiovascular disease.

Results of multiple prospective and case control studies have shown that patients with a moderately elevated plasma homocysteine concentration are more likely to develop venous and arterial thrombosis compared to the control population. Homocysteine seems to promote atherothrombosis by a variety of mechanisms. The precise pathogenic mechanism remains to be confirmed and it is not yet clear whether homocysteine itself or a related metabolite or a cofactor is primarily responsible for the atherothrombogenic effects of hyperhomocysteinemia. However, recent studies indicate that lowering an elevated homocysteine level does decrease the risk of atherosclerosis and blood clots. Until this issue has been more clearly defined, it appears prudent to make an effort to try to lower one's homocysteine levels through supplementation with B vitamins, which is an efficient and safe way to reduce an elevated homocysteine levels.

The MTHFR mutations appear to be medically irrelevant, as long as an individual's homocysteine level is normal. Therefore, it should be first the homocysteine level, not the MTHFR genetic status, to be tested in patients with or at risk for blood clots, atherosclerosis, or pregnancy complications.

It is well estabilished that healthly lifestyle lowers homocysteine concentrations. So the most important in everyday life is awareness that the level of homocysteine in blood is strongly influenced by several lifestyle factors such as nutrition, stress, smoking cigarettes, alcohol consumption, or physical inactivity. And therefore, exercise is a commonly recommended lifestyle intervention for individuals at risk for, or diagnosed with, cardio vascular disease. More specifically, we suggest that exercise, mild in aged people, but especially heavy physical activity, exerts its most favorable effect in subjects with hyperhomocysteinemia.

8. Acknowledgement

The authors wish to thank Dr. Cécil J.W. Meulenberg for proofreading and useful suggestions.

9. References

Barak AJ, Beckenhauer HC, Hidiroglou N, Camilo ME, Selhub J &Tuma DJ. (1993). The relationship of ethanol feeding to the methyl folate trap. *The Journal of alcoholism*, Vol.10, No.6, (1993), pp. 495-497, ISSN: 0021-8685.

Butz LWV & du Vigneaud V. (1932). The formation of a homologue of cystine by the decompensation of methionine with sulfuric acid. *Journal of Biological Chemistry*, Vol.99, pp. 135-142, ISSN 0021-9258.

Bolander-Gouaille C. (2001). *Focus on Homocysteine,* Springer-Verlag France, ISBN 2287596828, Berlin (etc).

Blount BC, Mack MM, Wehr CM, Mac Gregor JT, Hiatt RA Wang G, Wickramasinghe SN , Everson RB & Ames BN. (1997). Folate deficiency causes uracil misincorporation into human DNA and chromosome breakage: Implications for cancer and neuronal damage. *Proceedings of the National Academy of Sciences of the United States of America*, Vol.94, No.7, (1997), pp. 3290-3295, ISSN: 1091-6490.

Carey MC, Fennelly JJ & Fitz Gerald 0. (1968). Homocystinuria II. Subnormal serum folate levels, increased folate clearance and effects of folic acid therapy. *American Journal of Medicine*, Vol.45, (1997), pp. 26, ISSN: 0002- 9343.

Carson N & Neill DW. (1962). Metabolic abnormalities detected in a survey of mentally backward individuals in Northern Ireland. *Archives of Disease in Childhood*, Vol.37, (1962) pp. 505-513, ISSN: 00039888.

Cattaneo M. Hyperhomocysteinemia and Venous Thromboembolism. (2006). *Seminar in Thromobosis and Hemostasis*, Vol.32, No.7, (2006), pp. 716-723, ISSN: 0094-6176.

Dalton ML, Gadson PFJr, Wrenn RW & Rosenquist TH. (1997). Homocysteine signal cascade: production of phospholipids, activation of protein kinase C, and the induction of c-fos and c-myb in ssmooth muscle cells. *Federation of American Societies for Experimental Biology*, Vol.11, (1997), pp. 703-711, ISSN:0892-6638.

David R, Zamgwill L, Badarna M & Yassur Y. (1988). Epidemiology of retinal vein occluson and its association with glaucoma and increased intraocular pressure. *Ophthalmologica*, Vol. 197, (1988), pp. 69-74, ISSN: 0030-3755.

Dasarathy J, Gruca LL, Bennett C, Parimi PS, Duenas C, Marczewski S, Fierro JL & Kalhan SC. (1998). Methionine metabolism in human pregnancy. Current Opininion of Hematology, Vol.5, No.5, (1988), pp. 343-349, ISSN: 1065-6251.

De Bree A, Van Dusseldorp M, Brouwer IA, Van het Hof KH & Steegers- Theunissen RPM. (1997). Folate intake in Europe: recommended, actual and desired intake. *European Journal of Clinical Nutrition*; Vol.51, (1997), pp. 643-660, ISSN: 0954-3007.

Dinesh-K, K. (2004). Homocysteine and Cardiovascular Disesase. *Current Atherosclerosis Reports*, Vol.6, (2004), pp.101-106, ISSN: 1523-3804.

Falanga A, Ofosu FA, Cortelazzo S, Delaini F, Consonni R, Caccia R, Longatti S, Maran D, Rodeghiero F, Pogliani E, et al.(1993). Preliminary study to identify cancer patients at high risk of venous thrombosis following major surgery. *British Journal of Haematology*, Vol.85, No.4, (1993), pp. 745-750, ISSN: 0007-1048.

Fodinger M, Horl WH & Sunder-Plassmann G. (2000). Molecular biology of 5,10-methylenetetrahydrofolate reductase. *Journal of Nephrology*, Vol.13, (2000), pp. 20-33, ISSN: 1121-8428.

Gatt A & Markis M. Hyperhomocysteinemia and Venous Thrombosis. (2007). *Seminars in Hematology*, Vol. 44, (2007), pp. 70-76, ISSN: 00371963.

Gatt A, Makris A, Cladd H, Burcombe RJ, Smith JM, Cooper P, Thompson D & Makris M. (2007). Hyperhomocysteinemia in women with advanced breast cancer. *International Journal of Laboratory Hematology*, Vol.29, No.6, (2008), pp.421-425, ISSN:1751 -5521.

Godin CS & Crooks PA. (1986). In vitro inhibition of histamine metabolism in guinea pig lung by S-(-)-nicotine. *Journal of Pharmaceutical Sciences*, Vol.75, No.10, (1986), pp.945-95, ISSN: 0022-3549.

Graham IM, Daly LE, Refsum HM, Robinson K, Brattström LE, Ueland PM, Palma-Reis RJ, Boers GH, Sheahan RG, Israelsson B, Uiterwaal CS, Meleady R, McMaster D, Verhoef P, Witteman J, Rubba P, Bellet H, Wautrecht JC, de Valk HW, Sales Lúis AC, Parrot-Rouland FM, Tan KS, Higgins I, Garcon D, Andria G, et al. (1997). The European Concerted Action Project. *Journal of the American Medical Association*, Vol. 227, (1997), pp.1775-1781, ISSN: 00987484.

Hankey GJ & Eikelboom JW. (1999). Homocysteine and vascular disease. *Lancet*, Vol.354, No.9176, (1999), pp. 407-413, ISSN: 0140-6736.

Hultberg B, Andersson A & Sterner G. (1993). Plasma homocysteine in renal failure. *Clinical Nephrology*, Vol.40, (1993), pp. 223-235, ISSN: 0301- 0430.

Hultberg B, Andersson A & Isaksson A. (1997). The effects of homocysteine and copper ions on the concentration and redox status of thiols in cell line cultures. *Clinica Chimica Acta*, Vol.262, No.1-2,(1997), pp.39-51, ISSN: 0009-8981.

Janssen MC, den Heijer M, Cruysberg JR, Wollersheim H & Bredie SJ. (2005). Retinal vein occlusion: A form of venous thrombosis or a complication of atherosclerosis? A meta- analysis of thromophilic factor. *Journal of Thrombosis and Haemostasis*, Vol.93, (2005), pp. 1021-1026, ISSN: 1538-7933.

Koch HG, Nabel P, Junker R, Auberger K, Schobess R & Homberger A. (1999). The 677T genotype of the common MTHFR thermolabile variant and fasting homocysteine in childhood venous thrombosis. *European Journal of Pediatrics*, Vol.158, (1999), pp.113-116, ISSN: 0340- 6199.

Köktürk N, Kanbay A, Aydogdu M, Ozyilmaz E, Bukan N & Ekim N. (2010). Hyperhomocysteinemia Prevalence Among Patients with Venous Thromboembolism. *Clinical and applied thrombosis/hemostasis*, (August 2010), doi: 10.1177/1076029610378499. ISSN: 1076-0296

Kosch A, Koch HG, Heinecke A, Kurnik k, Heller C & Nowak-Gottl U. (2004). Increased fasting total homocysteine plasma levels as a risk factor for thromboembolism in children. *Journal of Thrombosis and Haemostasis*, Vol.91, (2004), pp. 308-314, ISSN: 1538-7933.

Lentz SR. (1998). Mechanisms of thrombosis in hyperhomocysteinemia. *Current Opinion in Hematology*, Vol.5, No.5 (1998), pp.309-359, ISSN: 1065-6251

MCCully KS. (1969). Vascular pathology of homocysteinemia: implications for pathogenesis of arteriosclerosis. *American Journal of Pathology*, Vol.56, (1969), pp. 111-128, ISSN: 00029440.

Meshkin B & Blum K. (2007). Folate Nutrigenetics: A Convergence of Dietary Folate Metabolism, Folic Acid Supplementation, and Folate Antagonist Pharmacogenetics. *Drug Metabolism Letters*, Vol.1, (2007), pp. 55-60, ISSN: 18723128.

Miller DR, Specker BL, Ho ML & Norman EJ. (1991). Vitamin B12 status in macrobiotic community. *American Journal of Clinical Nutrition*, Vol.53, (1991), pp.524-529. ISSN: 1938-3207.

Moat SJ, Lang D, McDowell IF, Clarke ZL, Madhavan AK, Lewis MJ & Goodfellow J. (2004). Folate, Homocysteine, Endothelial function and Cardiovascular disease. *Journal Nutritional Biochemistry*, Vol.15, No.2, (2004), pp. 64-79, ISSN: 09552863.

Moll S. (2004). Homocysteine, 10.07.2011, Availbale from: <Http://www.fvleiden.org/ask/77.html>.

Mudd SH, Edwards WA, Loeb PM, Brown MS & Laster L. (1970). Homocystinuria due to cystathionine synthase deficiency: the effect of pyridoxine. *Journal of Clinical Investigation*, Vol.49, (1970), pp. 1762, ISSN: 00219738.

Mudd SH, Skovby F, Levy HL, Pettigrew KD, Wilcken B, Pyeritz RE, Andria G, Boers GHJ, Bromberg IL, Cerone R, Fowler B, Grobe H, Schmidt H & Schweitzer L. (1985). The natural hystory of homocystinuria due to cystathionine beta-synthase deficiency. *The American Journal of Human Genetics,* Vol.37, No.1, (1985), pp.1-33, ISSN: 0002-9297.

Nishio E & Watanabe Y. (1997). Homocysteine as a modulator of plateled- derived growth factor action in vascular smooth muscle cells: a possible role for hydrogen peroxide. *British Journal of Pharmacology*, Vol.122, (1997), pp. 269-274, ISSN: 1476-5381.

Nygård O, Vollset SE, Refsum H, Stensvold I, Tverdal A, Nordrehaug JE, Ueland M & Kvåle G. (1995). Total plasma homocysteine and cardiovascular risk profile. The Hordaland Homocysteine Study, *Journal of the American Medical Association,* Vol. 274, No.19, (1995), pp. 1526-1533, ISSN: 00987484.

Nygård O, Nordrehaug JE, Refsum H, Ueland PM, Farstad M & Vollset SE. (1997a). Plasma homocysteine levels and mortality in patients with coronary artery disease. *The New England Journal of Medicine*, Vol. 337, No.4, (1997), pp. 230-236, ISSN: (1997a), ISSN:1533-4406.

Nygård O, Refsum H, Ueland PM, Stensvold I, Nordrehaug JE, Kvåle G & Vollset SE. (1997b). Coffee consumption and plasma total homocysteine: The Hordaland Homocysteine Study. *The American Journal of Clinical Nutrition*, Vol.65. No. 1, (1997), pp.136-143, ISSN: 0002-9165.

Pennypacker LC, Allen RH, Kelly JP, Matthews LM, Grigsby J, Kaye K, Lindenbaum J & Stabler SP.(1992). High prevalence of cobalamin deficiency in elderly outpatients. *The Journal of the American Geriatrics Society*, Vol. 40, No. 12, (1992), pp. 1197-1204, ISSN: 0002-8614.

Pettersson T, Friman C, Abrahamsson L, Nilsson B & Norberg B. (1998). Serum homocysteine and methylmalonic acid in patients with rheumatoid arthritis and cobalaminopenia. *Journal of Rheumatology*, Vol.25, (1998), pp. 859-863, ISSN: 1499-2752.

Perry TL, Hansen S, Love LD, Crawford LE & Tischler B. (1968). Tretament of homocystinuria with a low- methionine diet, supplemental cysteine and a methyl donor. *Lancet*, Vol.292, No.7566, (1968), pp. 474 – 478. ISSN: 0140-6736.

Pietrzik P& Brönstrup A. (1998). Vitamins B12, B6 and folate as determinants of homocysteine concentration in the healthy population. *European Journal of Pediatrics*, Vol.157, No.2, (1998), pp. S135-S138. ISSN: 1432-1076.

Plazar N. Jurdana M & Pišot R. (2008). The effect of 35-day bed rest on plasma homocysteine concentration. *Farmacevtski vestnik*, Vol.59, No.6, (2008), pp. 319-322, ISSN: 0014-8229.

Rickles FR, Levine M & Edwards RL. (1992). Hemostatic alteration in cancer patients. *Cancer and Metastasis Review*, Vol.11, (1992), pp. 237-248, ISSN: 1573-7233.

Ridker PM, Manson JE, Buring JE, Shih J, Matias M & Hennekens CH. (1999). Homocysteine and risk of cardiovascular disease among postmenopausal women. *Journal of the American Medical Association*, Vol.281, (1999), pp. 1817-1821, ISSN: 0098748.

Schriver RC, Beaudet AL, Sly WS & Valle D. (1995). *The metabolic and molecular basis of inherited disease*, Mc-Graw-Hill, ISBN 0-07-105432-4 New York. P. 1276-1319.

Silaste ML, Rantala M, Sämpi M, Alfthan G, Ato A & Kasänieiemi A. (2001). Polimorphisms of key enzymes in homocysteine metabolism affect diet responsiveness of plasma homocysteine in healthy women. *Journal of Nutrition*; Vol.131, (2001), pp. 2643-2647, ISSN: 0022-3166.

Stanger O, Herrmann W, Pietrzik K, Flower B, Geisel J, Dierkes J & Weger M. (2003). DACHLIGA Homocystein (German, Austrian and Swiss Homocysteine Society): Consensus paper on the regional clinical use of homocysteine, folic acid and B-vitamins in cardiovascular and thrombotic diseases: guidelines and recommendations. *Clinical Chemistry and Laboratory Medicine*, Vol.41, (2003), pp. 1392-13403, ISSN: 1434-6621.

Sun CF, Haven TR, Wu TL, Tsao KC & Wu JT. (2002). Serum total homocysteine increases with the rapid proliferation rate of tumor cells and decline upon cell death: a potential new tumor marker. *Clinica Chimica Acta*, Vol. 321, (2002), pp: 55-62., ISSN: 0009-8981.

Trosseau A. (1865). Phlegmasia alba dolens. *Clinique médicale de l'Hôtel-Dieu de Paris*, Vol.3, (1865), pp.654-712. ISBN-10: 0543873021.

Ulvike A, Vollset SE, Hoff G & Ueland PM. (2008). Coffee consumption and circulating B-vitamins in healthy middle-aged men and women. *Clinical Chemistry*, Vol.54, No.9, (2008), pp.1489-1496, ISSN: 0009-9147.

Ubbink JB, van dr Merwe A, Vermaak WJH & Delport R. (1993). Hyperhomocysteinemia and the response to vitamin supplementation. *Journal of Clinical Investigation*, Vol.71, (1993), pp. 993-998, ISSN: 0021-9738.

Ubbnik JB, Vermaak WHJ, van der Merwe A, Becker PJ, Delport R & Potgieter HC. (1994). Vitamin requierments for the treatment of hyperhomocysteinemia in humans. *Journal of Nutrition*, Vol.124, pp. 1927-1933, ISSN: 0022-3166.

Varga EA, Sturm AC, Misita CP & Moll S. (2005). Homocysteine and MTHFR Mutations: relation to Thrombosis and Coronary Artery Disease. *Circulation*, Vol.111, (2005), pp. 289-293, ISSN: 0009-7322.

Watanabe F, Abe K, Fujita T, Goto M, Hiemori M & Nakano Y. (1998). Effects of microwave heating on the loss of vitamin B12 in foods. *Journal Agricolture Food Chemistry*, Vol.46, No.1, (1998), pp. 206–210, ISSN: 0021-8561.

Weisberg IS, Park E, Ballman KV, Berger P, Nunn M, Suh DS, et al. (2003). Investigations of a common genetic variant in betaine-homocystein methyltransferase (BHMT) in coronary artery disease. *Atherosclerosis*, Vol.167, (2003), pp. 205-214, ISSN: 0021-9150.

Wilcken DE & Wilcken B. (1967). The pathogenesis of coronary artery disease. A possible role for methionine metabolism. *Journal of Clinical Investigation*, Vol.57, (1967), pp. 1079-1082, ISSN: 0021-9150.

Section 2

Venous Thromboembolism in Certain Groups of Patients

Venous Thromboembolism in Neonates, Children and Patients with Chronic Renal Disease - Special Considerations

Pedro Pablo García Lázaro[1], Gladys Patricia Cannata Arriola[2], Gloria Soledad Cotrina Romero[3] and Pedro Arauco Nava[3]
[1]Hospital Nacional Almanzor Aguinaga Asenjo, City of Chiclayo,
[2]Hospital Cayetano Heredia, City of Piura,
[3]Hospital Nacional Almanzor Aguinaga Asenjo, City of Chiclayo,
Perú

1. Introduction

1.1 Venous thromboembolism in neonates

Among children, the group of critically ill newborns presents the largest of population that suffering from thromboembolism. Making decisions regarding therapeutic strategies a challenge for the intensive care physician as the clinical significance of neonatal thrombosis varies from asymptomatic incidents to life or limb threatening events and, moreover, appropriate evidence-based treatment algorithms are lacking.

This review focuses on the incidence, pathophysiology, risks factors, diagnosis and treatment of venous thromboembolism in neonates

1.2 Incidence

The incidence of thromboembolic events in the pediatric age group is highest in neonates and infants <1 year of age (Monagle et al., 2008). Much of the published data regarding the epidemiology of neonatal venous thromboembolism (VTE) has come from national registry studies. The Canadian registry (Schmid & Andrew, 1995) reported 97 cases of wich 64 (66%) had venous involvement. The German neonatal registry (Nowak-Gottl et al., 1997) reported 79 cases of symptomatic thrombosis, including stroke. VTE accounted for 76% of cases. The overall incidence of symptomatic events was 0.51 per 10,000 births.

Male and female infants are affected with equal frecuency with the exception of renal vein thrombosis, which has a male predominance for unclear reasons (Chalmers, 2006).

1.3 Pathophysiologic

We must consider the multiple additive factors that contribute to the development of thromboembolism in neonates. Also, the hemostatic system of neonates is significantly different from that of children and adults (Veldman, 2008).

On the pro-coagulant side, especially the vitamin K-dependent coagulation factors (II, VII, IX, and X) and the components of the contact system (FIX,FXII, prekallkreine and high molecular weight kininogen) show significantly reduced plasma activities in neonates compared to children and adults. However, the vitamin K-dependent inhibitors of coagulation, protein C and protein S, are also reduced, counterbalancing the reduced clotting potential of neonatal plasma. In fact, both antithrombin and protein C concentrantions are decreased to approximately 30% of adults values in term and even lower in preterm newborns. Neonatal platelets have been reported to be hypo-reactive; however, this deficiency seems to be balanced by increased von Willebrand factor activity, resulting in overall normal platelet function (Veldman, 2008).

The activity of the fibrinolityc system in the newborn is reduced compared to adults and older children due to both decreased plasma activity of plasminogen and increased plasma levels of plasminogen activator inhibitor (PAI). The latter fact may explain the high rate of thromboembolic event (TE) associated with intravascular devices in newborns. However, to date there is no evidence that the neonatal hemostatic system either protects from or promotes thrombus formation. Of course, additional risk factors, eg, critical illness or congenital thrombophilia, have to be considered separately from the immaturity of neonatal hemostasis (Veldman, 2008). Given the siginificant differences between the plasma factor concentrations in different age groups, a detailed knowledge on the development of hemostasis is critical for the intensivist in order to adapt pharmacological approaches and interpret results from laboratory tests in the neonate with TE (Ignjatovich et al,. 2006; Ignjatovich et al,. 2007).

1.4 Risk factors

Neonatal VTE is frecuently associated with presence of significant underlying risk factors. As in older children central venous lines (CVLs) are the single most important contributing factor. Excluding cases of renal vein thrombosis (RVT), CVLs-related thrombosis accounted for 89% and 94% of VTE in the Canadian and Dutch registries, respectively (Schmidt and Andrew, 1995; van Ommen et al., 2001). These events involve the large vessels most frequently used for catheterization including the umbilical vein. Neonatal VTE related to the use of the umbilical venous catheter (UVC) has been the subject of studies involving sequential imaging. Using venography, Roy et al.,1997 documented UVC-associated thrombosis in 14 of 48 neonates (29%). As in older children, many of these events were asymptomatic and the incidence of thrombosis was highly dependent on the imaging modality used (Chalmers, 2006).

Critical illness is a well-recognized risk factor for TE in all age groups. Inmobilization, rapid changes in intravascular volume and extensive intravascular instrumentation contribute to the enhanced risk of venous and arterial thrombosis in patients in intensive care units. (Veldman, 2008). Additional risk factors include, but are not limited to, asphyxia, maternal diabetes, poor cardiac output and dehydration. Neonates are born with a high hematocrit and tend to contract their intravascular volume within the first days of life, making them even more prone to thromboembolic events (Veldman, 2008).

In the neonatal population, sepsis is particularly devastating, as it causes 45% of late deaths in the neonatal intensive care unit (NICU). Neonates with sepsis develop an acquired pro-thrombotic state due to increased consumption of already limited supplies of coagulation inhibitors. Furthermore, plasma activity of plasminogen activator inhibitor (PAI) is increased in sepsis and levels of protein C are reduced. The latter fact has been reported to correlate with poor outcomes in adults and neonates. Ongoing consumption of coagulation factors and platelets resulting in microcirculatory thrombosis likely contributes to sepsis-induced multi-organ failure and death. Macro-circulatory thrombotic events are rare in this setting but can occur, especially in babies who have arterial umbilical catheters (UACs) or UVCs in situ (Veldman, 2008).

Turebylu., 2007 reported that congenital thrombophilia not to be associated with UVC thrombosis. Revel-Vilk et al., 2003 reported that in neonates inherited prothrombotic coagulation proteins do not contribute significantly to the pathogenesis of venous TEs; they concluded that the most siginificant aetiological risk factors are the presence of a central venous line and other medical conditions.

Heller et al., 2000 reported an elevated odds ratio for the presence of congenital thrombophilia in neonates with renal, portal or hepatic venous thrombosis and recommended that neonates with TE should undergo an extensive screening, included resistance to activated protein C (APC-R), protein C, protein S, antithrombin activity, activities of coagulation factors VIIIC and XII, lipoprotein-A, histidine-rich glycoprotein, heparin cofactor II, antiphospholipid antibodies, lupus anticoagulants, as well as fasting homocysteine concentrations. In addition, DNA-based assays (factor V G1691A mutation or factor V Leiden, factor II G20210A variant and MTHFR C677T genotype) should be considered. Whereas DNA-based mutation analysis can be performed at any time point, protein-based assays should not be carried out in the first 6-8 months after the event and oral anticoagulation is recommended to be discontinued at 14-30 days before plasma samples for thrombophilia diagnosis are drawn.

Deficiency of one of the important hemostasis control proteins, protein C, protein S or antithrombin, occurs less frequently, but results in a more potent prothrombotic state. Heterozygous deficiency of these proteins is difficult to diagnose in the newborn period, because the neonatal levels are much lower than the adult reference range. Homozygous deficiency of Protein C or S typically presents in the perinatal period with significant thrombosis resulting in purpura fulminans. Compoud heterozygosity of one of the natural anticoagulants in association with Factor V Leiden may cause a similar clinical picture (Beardsley, 2007).

1.5 Diagnosis

1.5.1 Clinical

Intravascular catheters are responsible for more than 80% of venous thrombotic complications.Signs and symptoms of catheter-related thrombosis vary from diminished blood flow through the cateter to tenderness and swelling of the affected extremity or swelling of the neck and head associated with superior vena cava syndrome. Although clinically apparent thrombi occur in less than 5% of neonates with a central line. (Beardsley, 2007).

Renal vein thrombosis (RVT) is the most common form of non-catheter-related thrombosis (Nathan et al., 2003). Risk factors for RVT include maternal diabetes, dehydration, infection, asphyxia, polycythemia, prematurity,critical illness, femoral CVL and male gender (chest,913,veldman). Approximately 80% present within the first month and usually within the first week of life and it is likely that a number of these :events initially develop antenatally. (Monagle et al., 2008; Veldman, 2008). Presenting symptoms and clinical findings are different in neonates and older patients and are influenced by the extent and rapidity of thrombus formation. Neonates usually have a flank mass, hematuria, proteinuria, thrombocytopenia and nonfunction of the involved kidney. (Nathan et al., 2003). Approximately 25% of cases are bilateral and 52-60% are reported to have evidence of extension into the inferior vena caval (IVC). (Monagle et al., 2008). Overall survival following neonatal RVT is generally favorable. Four small cohort studies with variable follow-up reported 81-100% of neonates survived. Clinical sequelae included chronic renal impairment and hypertension. (Monagle et al., 2008)

Thombosis of the inferior vena cava can present with signs resembling obstruction of the renal vein (hematuria and retroperitoneal mass); however, these will occur bilaterally when the inferior vena cava is affected. In addition, the lower limbs may be edematous and, if blood flow is susbstantially impared, the child may be in respiratory distress and may have high blood pressure. (Veldman, 2008)

Signs of impared liver function, hepatomegaly and splenomegaly should raise the suspicion of portal vein thrombosis (PVT); however, only about 10% of children with PVT develop acute clinical symptoms (Veldman, 2008).

1.5.2 Imaging

The echocardiography or abdominal ultrasound is the most commonly applied diagnostic method to confirm clinical suspicion of TE or to screen babies for clinically silent disease. (Roy et al, 2002) comparing echocardiographic investigations with venograms and reported a sensitivity of 21-43% and specificities ranging from 76-94%. This study concluded that venography is required to accurately diagnose UVC related TE in neonates.

1.5.3 Laboratory

Initial laboratory work-up in a neonate in whom thrombosis is suspected should include a full blood count as well as a coagulation screening with determination of prothrombin time, thrombin time and activated partial thromboplastin time.

D-dimers are a positive finding in almost all critically ill neonates. Conversely, negative D-dimers are relatively accurate in ruling out thrombosis in most patients, including neonates.

In almost all neonates, platelet numbers decrease after birth. However, a sudden and severe drop in platelet counts should alert the intensivist. The thrombocytopenia remains one of the most sensistive indicators for micro- (in the setting of sepsis) or macro-circulatory thrombosis (Veldman, 2008).

Also it has been recommended that infants who are diagnosed with clinically significant VTE should undergo testing for inherited and acquired thrombophilic traits. (Beardsley, 2007).

1.6 Management

There are no published randomized controlled trials (RCTs) and no large cohort studies that report on the outcomes of different treatment modalities in the management of neonatal

VTE. Valuable and comprehensive evidence-based clinical practice guidelines have been developed by the American College of Chest Physicians (ACCP) on antithrombotic therapy in neonates and children (Monagle et al, 2008). Their recommendations are necessarily based on extrapolation of principles of therapy from adult guidelines, limited clinical information from registries, individual case studies and knowledge of current common clinical practice.

The following is the summary of the recommendations of the ACCP 2008 on Anticoagulation and Trombolytic Therapy for neonates with VTE: We suggest that central venous lines (CVL) or UVCs associated with confirmed thrombosis be removed, if possible, after 3 to 5 days of anticoagulation (Grade 2C).It is a weak recommendation. We suggest either initial anticoagulation, or supportive care with radiologic monitoring (Grade 2C); however, we recommend subsequent anticoagulation if extension of the thrombosis occurs during supportive care (Grade 1B). It is a strong recommendation. We suggest anticoagulation should be with either of the following: (1) LMWH given bid and adjusted to achieve an anti-FXa level of 0.5–1.0 U/mL: or (2) UFH for 3 to 5 days adjusted to achieve an anti-FXa of 0.35 to 0.7 U/mL or a corresponding APTT range, followed by LMWH. We suggest a total duration of anticoagulation of between 6 weeks and 3 months (Grade 2C). We suggest that if either a CVL or a UVC is still in place on completion of therapeutic anticoagulation, a prophylactic dose of LMWH be given to prevent recurrent VTE until such time as the CVL or UVC is removed (Grade 2C). We recommend against thrombolytic therapy for neonatal VTE unless major vessel occlusion is causing critical compromise of organs or limbs (Grade 1B). We suggest that if thrombolysis is required the clinician use tPA and supplement with plasminogen fresh frozen plasma) prior to commencing therapy (Grade 2C). For neonates or children with unilateral renal vein thrombosis (RVT) in the absence of renal impairment or extension into the inferior vena cava, we suggest supportive care with monitoring of the RVT for extension or anticoagulation with UFH/LMWH or LMWH in therapeutic doses; we suggest continuation for 3 months (Grade 2C). For unilateral RVT that extends into the inferior vena cava, we suggest anticoagulation with UFH/LMWH or LMWH for 3 months (Grade 2C). For bilateral RVT with various degrees of renal failure, we suggest anticoagulation with UFH and initial thrombolytic therapy with TPA, followed by anticoagulation with UFH/LMWH (Grade 2C).Remark: LMWH therapy requires careful monitoring in the presence of significant renal impairment.

2. Venous thromboembolism and chronic kidney disease

Pulmonary embolism and Deep Vein Thrombosis are a wide spectrum of a single disease defined as Venous Thromboembolism, and it occurs for the first time in approximately 100 persons per 100,000 each year in the United States and rises exponentially from less than 5 cases per 100,000 persons at 15 years and less to approximately 500 cases per 100,000 persons at age 80 years (White, 2003; Ageno, 2006; Heit, 2008).

An understanding of the risk factors for venous thrombosis is necessary in order to increase the prevention of this disease in high risk individuals and groups of patients.

The major risk factors for thrombosis include endogenous pattern characteristics like obesity and genetic factors, and triggering factors such as surgery, immobility or pregnancy. Venous thrombosis tends to occur due to additive effects of endogenous, genetic and environmental risk factors present simultaneously (Cushman, 2007).

Chronic kidney disease is common in the general population, affecting 13% of adults in the United States between 1999 and 2004 (Coresh 2007).

There are several questions about the relation between venous thromboembolism and chronic kidney disease. Is the chronic kidney disease a risk factor for venous thromboembolism? What are the mechanisms involved in these diseases? And finally how to treat these patients?

2.1 Epidemiology of thromboembolism associated to chronic kidney disease

2.1.1 Chronic kidney disease and venous thromboembolism

There are few prospective studies about this association, with this objective and using the data from the Longitudinal Investigation of Thromboembolism Etiology Study, 19,073 middle-aged and elderly adults were categorized on the basis of the determination of the glomerular flltration rate and cystatin C (data avalaible in 4,734 participants). During a mean follow up time of 11.8 years, 413 participants developed venous thromboembolism (41 % idiopathic and 59% secondary). Compared with the participants with normal kidney function, the relative risk for venous thromboembolism was 1.28 (95% confidence interval) for those with mildly decrease kidney function and 2.09 for those with stage 3 or 4 of chronic kidney disease. The authors concluded that middle -age and elderly patients with chronic kidney disease stages 3 through 4 evidence all increased risk for incident venous thromboembolism, suggesting that prophylaxis may **be** particularly important in this population (Wattanakit, 2008).

Similar results were reported by Folsom et al, in a prospective cohort of 10,700 patients, in whom estimated the glomerular filtration rate from prediction equations based on serum creatinine or cystatin C, and follow up for the occurrence of venous thromboembolism for over a median of 8.3 years. The adjusted hazard ratios of total venous thromboembolism and estimated glomerular filtration rate based in cystatin C was 1.0 for normal kidney function, 1.4 for mildly impaired renal function and 1.94 for stage 3 and 4 of chronic kidney disease, these hazard ratios were moderately attenuated to 1.0, 1.26 and 1.6 respectively with adjustment for hormone replacement therapy, diabetes and body mass index. Association between chronic kidney disease, based on estimated glomerular filtration rate using cystatin C, and venous thromboembolism were slightly stronger for idiopathic venous thromboembolism than for secondary venous thromboembolism. In contrast, creatinine glomerular filtration rate was no associate with total venous thromboembolism occurrence.(Foslom, 2010).

Another prospective cohort study 8,495 subjects whit chronic kidney disease stages 1 to 3 in which renal function and albuminuria were assessed, they concluded that stages 1 or 2 of chronic kidney disease are risk factors for venous thromboembolism in presence of albuminuria, and the risk of venous thromboemboslim is more related to albuminuria than to impaired glomerular filtration rate (Ocak 2010).

2.1.2 End-stage renal disease and venous thromboembolism

Independent of co-morbidity chronic dialysis patients have high risk for pulmonary embolism, in 1996 in the United States, the overall incidence rate of pulmonary embolism was 149.9/100,000 dialysis patients, compared with 24.6/100,000 persons in the general population. In this study the younger dialysis patients had the greatest relative risk for pulmonary embolism (Tveit, 2002). Similar results by Allen et al, that showed an incidence of 8.3% of venous thromboembolism in dyalisis patiens (Allen, 1987).

2.1.3 Nephrotic syndrome and venous thromboembolism

Several studies consider Nephrotic Syndrome as a risk factor for venous thromboembolism. In one of the largest studies, Kayali el al, studied 925,000 patients discharged from hospitals in the United States with the diagnosis of nephrotic syndrome, 0.5% had pulmonary embolism, 6.5% had deep vein thrombosis and less than 0.5% had renal vein thrombosis. The relative risk of pulmonary embolism (in patients with the nephrotic syndrome) was 1.39 and for deep vein thrombosis was 1.72. Among patients aged 18-39 years the relative risk of deep vein thrombosis increases to 6.81 (Kayali, 2008).

Another prospective study of 298 patients with nephrotic syndrome, with a mean follow up of 10±9 years, the annual incidence of venous thromboembolism was 1.02%, over the first 6 months of follow up; the rate of venous thromboembolism was 9.85. In this group of patients, proteinuria and serum albumin levels tended to be related to venous tromboembolism, however, only the predictive value of the ratio of proteinuria to serum albumin was significant but not the estimated glomerular filtration rate.(Bakhtawar, 2008)

For instance, estimated glomerular filtration rate using cystatin C, albuminuria and ratio proteinuria to serum albumin have predictive value for venous thromboembolism in patients with chronic renal disease.

2.1.4 Renal transplantation and venous thromboembolism

In renal transplantation, few studies had evaluated the risk of venous thromboembolism, the largest one used the United States Renal Data System database to study 28,924 patients receiving a kidney transplant, the rate of VTE occurring 1.5 to 3 years after transplantation was 2.9 episodes/1,000 person-years. Estimated glomerular filtration rate less than 30 mL/min/1.73 m2 versus higher at the end of the first year after renal transplantation was associated with significantly increased risk for later venous thromboembolism (adjusted hazard ratio, 2.05; 95% confidence interval, 1.08 to 3.89). Patients with severe chronic kidney disease, after renal transplantation should be regarded as high risk for late venous tromboembolism, which is a potentially preventable cause of death in this population (Abbott, 2004).

A prospective study of a cohort of 578 patients with renal transplantation, reports 9.1 % incidence of deep vein thrombosis of the lower limbs, 39.5% were asymptomatic and the diagnosis was made during routine ultrasound examination. Those patients, who experience venous thromboembolism, were at high risk of recurrence after thromboprophylaxis withdrawal (Poli, 2006).

Co-morbilities like diabetes mellitus could increase the risk of venous thromboembolism, in a prospective study the frequency of deep vein thrombosis during the first 3 weeks after kidney transplantation has been evaluated using the combination of thermography and strain-gauge plethysmography for objective diagnosis. 83 consecutive patients were included, 33 with juvenile diabetes mellitus. The overall frequency of thrombosis was 24.1%, diabetes mellitus being a significant risk factor (Bergqvist, 1985).

Epidemiological studies have attempted to define risk in terms of modifiable (drugs, dialysis modality, surgical procedure) and no modifiable (age, diabetes mellitus, vascular anomalies, factor or identify changes in coagulation or fibrinolysis) promoting a more thrombotic state. Most recently the evolution of thrombophilia research has established the potential for inherited hypercoagulability to predispose to acute allograft thrombosis. Inheritance of the factor V Leiden (FVL), prothrombin G20210A mutation, or the presence of antiphospholipid antibodies may increase the risk of renal allograft thrombosis certain 3-fold in selected patients. Patients with end-stage renal disease due to systemic lupus erythematosus appear at particularly high risk of thrombosis, especially if they have either antiphospholipid antibodies or detectable β2-glycoprotein-1. (Irish, 2004).

2.2 Mechanisms of venous thrombosis in patients with chronic kidney disease

The individual risk of venous thromboembolism varies as a result of a complex interaction between congenital and transient or permanent acquired risk factors.

Virchow summarized the pathophysiology of venous thromboembolism in his famous triad: venous stasis, endothelial damage and hypercoagulability (Ageno 2006 as cited in Virchow, 1856)

Stasis predisposes to venous thrombosis by reducing the clearance of activated coagulation factors, the mixing of this activated coagulation factors and inhibitors and the dilution of activated coagulation factors.

Vessel wall damage is more important in the pathogenesis of arterial thrombus. Venous endothelial damage results in endothelial cell detachment and exposure of blood to tissue factor and other subendothelial components that activate coagulation.

Hypercoagulable states could be in several situations: increase thrombin production following surgery or decrease activity of endogenous anticoagulants.

On the whole, venous thromboembolism probably has understood as a multicausal disease in which more than one genetic or environmental condition coincides to produce clinically apparent thrombosis (Rosendaal,1999).

2.2.1 Procoagulant markers

To elucidate the mechanisms that could increase the risk of venous thromboembolism in patients with chronic kidney diseases, some studies had investigated the levels of the procoagulant markers.

Patients with end stage renal disease and predialysis renal failures, nephrotic syndrome and mildly chronic kidney disease had elevated level of C Reactive Protein, fibrinogen, d-dimer, Factor VIII, Factor VII, and Von Willebrand, these high levels are due to increase synthesis out of proportion to urinary loss while lower levels of coagulation factors like IX, XI, and XII due to increased urinary loss (Keller, 2008; Vaziri, 1980). On the other hand, an association between increased levels of coagulation factors VIII, FIX and F XI and an increased risk of venous thromboembolism has been reported, the mechanisms and clinical significance of such association are still unclear (Crowther, 2003).

2.2.2 Decrease endogenous anticoagulants

In the nephrotic syndrome the hypercoagulable state is distinguished by an increase in coagulation factors (V, VIII and fibrinogen) a decrease in the levels of antitrombin III and S Proteins, an increase in alpha 2 antiplasmin activity and exaggerated platelet adhesiveness and aggregation. This prothrombotic state may be aggravated by additional rheological factors (immobilization, diuretic therapy, etc.) (Keusch, 1989; Adams, 2008).

The lower level of antithrombin III in patients with nephrotic syndrome is probably due to increased urinary loss.(Vaziri, 1984).

2.2.3 Platelet activation and aggregation

P-selectin is a marker of platelet activation and is increased in nephrotic syndrome patients. Platelet aggregation increases because of hypoalbuminemia that result in an increase avalaibility of thromboxane a-2 that is a potent platelet agonist (Jackson, 1982).

2.2.4 Reduced fibrinolysis

Fibrin cloths with reduced permeability, increased clot stiffness and reduced fibrinolysis susceptibility may predispose to thrombosis. Using permeability and turbidity studies in 22 end stage renal disease patients and 24 healthy controls. Fibrin clots made from plasma of patients with chronic renal disease were found to be less permeable, less compactable and less susceptible to fibrinolysis than clots from controls (Siøland, 2007).

Another study in 33 patiens in long term haemodialysis has demonstrated unfavorably altered clot properties that may be associated with increase cardiovascular mortality (Unaas, 2008) There are studies that demonstrates that individuals with reduced fibrinolytic potential as measured by plasma based assays , have an increased risk of developing a first venous thrombosis. Whether this hypofibrinolytic state determined by genetic or adquired factors or a combination of them and which proteins are evolved is at present unknow (Lisman, 2005).

In conclusion, chronic kidney disease patients presents a pro-thrombotic state that increases the risk of venous thromboembolism and comprises alteration of platelet functions, coagulation factors, endogenous anticoagulants and fibrinolytic system, many mechanism are still unknown and opens a potential field for investigation.

2.3 Treatment of venous thromboembolism in chronic renal disease patients

Anticoagulants are widely used to prevent and treat venous thromboembolism, these drugs are often used in patients with renal impairment. Renal impairment is at the same time, a risk factor for bleeding and thrombosis during anticoagulant therapy and may influence the balance between the safety and efficacy of such drugs (Harder, 2011).

The available anticoagulants for the treatment of thromboembolism are heparins, the Factor X inhibitor fondaparinux, warfarin and the new anticoagulants Factor X inhibitors and direct thrombin inhibitors. Most of the antithrombotics are eliminated primarily by the kidneys , so dosing in patients with several renal impairment may require dosage reduction or increase frequency of monitoring for bleeding and thromboembolism complications or both(Lobo, 2007).

Decisions for anticoagulation therapy respect the agent selected, dose, duration of treatment, and approaches to monitoring should balance the risks between bleeding and thrombosis.

2.3.1 Indirect thrombin Inhibitors

2.3.1.1 Unfractionated Heparin (UFH)

Heparin is a large, heterogeneous compound of approximately 45 saccharide units that indirectly binds to and increases the enzymatic activity of antithrombin III, against activated Factors II, and X. Unfractionated Heparin clearance is the result of a combination of rapid, saturable mechanism via the endothelium and the reticuloendothelial system in liver, and a slower, non saturable mechanism through the kidneys (Follea, 1987) However UFH remain the anticoagulant choice for in-hospital treatment of patients with thromboembolic disorders who also have renal dysfunction.

There are no recommendations from the American College of Chest Physicians (ACCP) Consensus Conference on Antithrombotic Therapy and from the manufacturers for dose reduction of UFH in patients with chronic renal impairment (Kearon, 2008). The monitoring of the activated partial thromboplastin time is recommended while UFH are administered to renal impairment patients.

In acute thromboembolic events, an intravenous bolus dose up to 80 units/kg may be administered, but in the absence of an emergent need for anticoagulation or high risk situations, the bolus dose could be omitted and just a continuous infusion may be initiated with the advantage of gradually establishing of the anticoagulation and limiting the risk of bleeding. Initial continuous infusion of unfractionated heparin do not require special adjustments because of chronic kidney disease alone and goal activated partial time of thromboplastin should be targeted to the indication for anticoagulant therapy. Another option is subcutaneous weight adjusted dosing. (Dager, 2010)

2.3.1.2 Low molecular weight heparin (LMWH)

Low molecular weight heparins may not be considered as the preferred option for initial parenteral anticoagulation in chronic kidney disease patients, but they could be considered in special situations because these agents are primarily eliminated on kidneys and dosing adjustments are needed as renal failure progresses (Kearon, 2006).

A meta analysis was performed to study the incidence of bleeding in chronic kidney disease patients treated with low molecular weight heparins like enoxaparin, dalteparin and tinzaparin. Enoxaparin has elevated levels of anti-factor Xa and an increased risk for mayor bleeding, suggesting empirical dose adjustment of enoxaparin in patients with severe renal impairment. In patients with mild to moderate renal impairment there are not required dose adjustment of enoxaparin [Lim, 2006]

For venous tromboembolism prophylactic doses of enoxaparin the American College of Chest Physicians (ACCP) recommendations for patients with severe renal impairment is to lower or halve the standard dose. For the treatment of venous thromboembolism in patients with severe renal impairment the ACCP guidelines recommended either using unfractionated heparin instead of low molecular weight heparins. No especific dose recommendations are made in this guidelines for other low molecular weight heparins in venous thromboembolism. For tinzaparin and dalteparin monitoring of anticoagulant activity in patients with renal failure should be considered.

2.3.1.3 Fondaparinux

Fondaparinux is a synthetic pentasaccharide, that inhibits factor Xa by binding to antithrombin. After subcutaneous administration the peak plasma concentration is achieved within 2 hours, the half life is 17 hours in young healthy subjects and 21 hours in the elderly. Up to 80% of fondaparinux is eliminated as unchanged drug via the kidneys.

However the ACCP guidelines for VTE prevention do not recommend specific doses adjustments for fondaparinux in renal impaired patients, depending of the circumstances the guidelines recommended avoiding the anticoagulant, lowering dose or monitoring anticoagulant activity [Hirsh,2008]

The summary of manufacturers insert states contraindicated of fondaparinux in patients with severe renal impairment (clearance of creatinine ‹20 ml/min) and use with caution in patients with moderate renal impairment (creatinine clearance 30 a 50 ml/min)[Harder 2011]

2.3.2 Vitamin K antagonists

Vitamin K antagonist inhibit the hepatic synthesis of factors II, VII, IX and X and protein C and S. There are various vitamina K antagonists, however, warfarin is the most commonly used around the world.

After oral administration warfarin is rapidly absorbed reaching the plasma peak concentration within 90 minutes, the peak therapeutic effect is acquired at 36 hours. Warfarin undergoes oxidative metabolism via the CYP450 system in the liver and less than 1% of the drug is excreted unchanged in the urine. (Ansell, 2008)

The risk of bleeding and thromboembolic complications is increased when using warfarin in the chronic kidney disease population and depends of the INR target, incidence of values outside of the target or other comorbid conditions. Warfarin dosing requirements tend to be lower as renal function declines. (Limdi , 2009) Concurrent drug interactions and acute medical problems such as heart failure or infections can influence the dose response to warfarin. Because the complexity of managing warfarin and increased risk of adverse outcomes in the chronic kidney disease setting, warfarin management in those patients should be referred when possible to dedicated anticoagulant services.(Dager ,2003).

2.3.3 Novel oral anticoagulants in patiens with renal disease

2.3.3.1 Dabigatran etexilate

Dabigatran etexilate is a direct thrombin inhibitor, currently approved for the prevention of venous thromboembolism in orthopedic surgery patients. After oral administration peak plasma concentrations are achieved within 2 hours of administration. Elimination of dabigatran is predominantly via the renal pathway, 80% of the administered dose is excreted unchanged in the urine within the first 24 hours after an intravenous dose and is contraindicated in patients with severe renal impairment (Stangier, 2008)

Limited data are avalaible on dabigatran pharmacokinetics in patients with renal impairment for venous thromboembolism treatment.(Dahl, 2009)

2.3.3.2 Rivaroxaban

Rivaroxaban inhibits both free and clot-bound Factor Xa, this oral anticoagulant has been approved for the prevention of venous thromboembolism after elective hip or knee replacement surgery in adults (Bauer, 2008)

Rivaroxaban has a dual mode of elimination hepatic and renal and the inhibition of factor Xa activityalso increased with the reduce renal function. Rivaroxaban is not recommended for patients with a Creatine clearance of less than 15 mil/min. (Kubitza, 2010). To the date there are not reported studies for rivaroxaban in patients with renal impairment for venous thromboembolism.

2.3.3.3 Apixaban

Apixaban inhibits both free and clot-bound factor Xa Apixaban is rapidly absorved in the stomach and small intestine, reaching peaks concentrations approximately 1 to 3 hours after oral administration. The elimination includes renal and biliary excretion, and the drug has a mean elimination half life of 8 to 15 hours. (Shantsila, 2008;Frost,2007)

There are limited data about the clearance of apixaban in patients with renal impairment.

In presence of heparin induced thrombocytopenia or antithrombin deficiency directs thrombin inhibitors may be options for anticoagulation. They are argatroban, bivalidurin and lepirudin, avalaible only by continous venous infusion or subcutaneous injection.

2.3.3.4 Argatroban

Argatroban is eliminated in liver and no adjustment in dosing is required for renal insufficiency or hemodyalisis, the mean dose in heparin induced thrombocytopenia was 1.6 µg/kg/min, targeting activated partial thromboplastin time 1.5 to 3.0 times control. In patients with renal failure it has been suggest lower dosing requirements with dose reduction of approximately 0.1 to 0.6 µg/kg/min for each 30 ml/min decrease in the creatinine clearance. (Hursting, 2008; Arpino, 2004)

2.3.3.5 Lepirudin

Lepirudin is the agent most dependent of renal elimination and requires significant dose reductions as renal function declines.

2.3.3.6 Bivalirudin

Bivalirudin is eliminated independent of renal function, with 80% removed enzimatically, it has also been observed to be removed by ultrafiltration. For patients with renal dysfunction and heparin induced thrombocytopenia, dose reductions has been suggested. The extend depends on the degree of renal dysfunction and form of renal replacement therapy. The target activated partial thromboplastin time for both lepirudin and bivalirudin is 1.5 to 2.5 times baseline and argatroban 1.5 to 3 times baseline, which may be different from the range specified for unfractionated heparin.(Dager, 2007; Kiser,2008).

In conclusion the unfractionated heparin continues been the anticoagulant of choice for chronic kidney disease patients, because it's short half life, reliable monitoring, reversibility and independence of renal function. Of the oral anticoagulants, warfarine is a safe alternative to unfractionated heparin, easy to monitor and does not requires dose alteration in chronic kidney disease.

Stage	Kidney damage	Glomerular filtration rate CrCl, mL/min/1.73m^2
1	Normal o Increased GFR	≥90
2	Mild decrease in GFR	60 to 80
3	Moderate decrease in GFR	30 to 59
4	Severe decrease in GFR	15 to 29
5	Kidney failure (End stage renal disease)	<15(or dialysis)

CrCl: creatinine clearance
[a] Clasification by National Kidney Foundation. Chronic kidney disease is defined as either kidney damage or GFR of <60 mL/min/1.73m2 for ≥ 3 months. Kidney damage is defined as pathological abnormalities or markers of damage, including abnormalities in blood or urine test or imaging studies.GFR reported by the National Kidney Foundation, using the modification of Diet in Renal Disease Study equation based on age, gender, race, and serum creatinine
[Reference: Harder, 2011]

Table 1. Clasification of Renal impairment

Anticoagulant	Elimination	Half life*	Monitoring	Antidote	Dose adjustment in severe renal impairment
UFH	RES,renal minimal	30-150 min after IV administration	aPTT, anti Xa ACT	Protamine	No dose adjustment Monitoring high doses
LMWH	Mainly renal RES minimal	2-8 h after SC administration	Anti Xa	Protamine partially effective	Yes
Bivalirudin	Proteolytic cleavage 80% Renal 20%	~25 min after IV administration	ACT	None	Yes
Argatroban	Hepatic 100%(CYP3A4)	40-50 min after IV administration	aPTT,ACT, ECT	None	No
Fondaparinux	Renal>80%	17 -21 h after SC administration	Anti Xa	None	Drug no recommended
Vitamin K agonists	Hepatic 100% (CYP2C9)	~36-42 h	INR	Vitamin K	Careful dose titration
Rivaroxaban	Renal 50% hepatic 50%	7 -11 h	Anti Xa	None	Not recommended
Dabigatran	Renal 80%	8 -10 h	ECT	None	Not recommended
Apixaban	Renal 50%	8 – 15 h	INR, aPTT, Anti Xa	None	Yes

ACT =Activated clotting time; aPTT=activated partial thromboplastin time; CYP= cytochrome p450 ECT = ecarin clotting time; INR= International normalized ratio; IV =Intravenous; LMWH= low molecular weight heparin; RES= reticuloendothelial system; SC= subcutaneous; UFH= unfractionated heparin. {Reference: Grand'Maison A, Charest A,Geerts W, 2005 ; Harder S,2011]

Table 2. Anticoagulants characteristics and dose adjustment in severe renal impairment

While low molecular weight heparins, fondaparinux and direct thrombin inhibitors may offer alternatives to unfractionated heparin in patients with chronic kidney disease, more evidence are needed to determine the safe dose and monitoring strategy.

3. Thrombosis in infants and children

Thromboembolism (TE) is still regarded as a rare event in childhood and therefore knowledge of diagnostics, therapy and prophylaxis is limited among general pediatricians. During the past years, however, it is increasingly recognized as having significant impact on mortality, chronic morbidity and the normal development of children, which has led to an enhanced sensitivity toward considering such events in respective patients. Besides the greater awareness, an objective increase in childhood thrombosis is due to the medical progress in the treatment of critically ill patients. This seemingly contradictory observation is easily explained by the increasing use of central catheters and innovative interventional procedures in the treatment of premature infants, neonates and older children who are critically ill, suffering from complex cardiac defects, and from malignant disease, respectively. Therapeutic and prophylactic measures have subsequently become increasingly important, but in addition to the complexity of the clinical background and the heterogeneity in the pattern of acquired and inherited risk factors for TE among patients, the physiological significant differences of the coagulation system between newborns, young children and adolescents and differences in drug metabolism do not allow general recommendations for therapeutic interventions like thrombolysis and prophylactic anticoagulation for the different clinical conditions. This situation is further complicated by a lack of availability of pediatric formulations and pediatric data for new drugs.

The increasing knowledge of exogenous and endogenous thrombophilic risk factors has initiated a number of studies to assess the impact of such factors with respect to their contribution to the thrombophilic state, both individually but also in concert with other factors. In addition to their impact on a first thrombotic event, much of the interest is now focused on their importance for thrombotic relapses. Only such studies will give us an answer to questions concerning the indications for treatment, prophylaxis and its optimal duration. All management recommendations are reflecting the authors' experiences and opinions and are not based on evidence gained by controlled trials as such trials are either completely lacking or still ongoing.

3.1 Epidemiology

The annual incidence of TE in childhood in general is considerably lower than in adults, with a reported frequency of 0.07 to 0.14 per 10.000 children or 5.3 per 10,000 referrals of children to the hospital. The results of a prospective German study suggested an incidence of 5.2 per 100,000 neonates, and a prospective Dutch study resulted in an estimate of 1.4 per 100,000 children and adolescents (Parasuraman & Goldhaber , 2006). More than 80% of TE in childhood were on a background of a severe preceding illness or other comparable predisposing factors. (Kuhle et al, 2004) Arterial TE in children is less common than venous thrombosis (Kuhle et al, 2004) with the exception of stroke. The estimated yearly incidence of stroke in childhood is between 3-8 per 100,000. (Giroud et al, 1995; Lynch et al, 2002). The highest incidence of 25-35 per 100,000 live births has been reported for neonates (Chalmer, 2005). In addition to its impact on the development of children, stroke also quantitatively plays the most important role.

The reasons for the lower incidences of TE in children compared to adults are not completely understood; an intact vascular endothelium, the lower capacity of thrombin generation (Haidi et al, 2006) and elevated levels of -2-macroglobulin, an inhibitor of thrombin, are possible age-dependent modifying factors in children. There are two age-related peaks in the frequency of thromboembolic disorders in children and adolescents: the first peak corresponds to the perinatal/neonatal period, with the highest relative incidence, and the second is observed post puberty in adolescents, with a higher frequency in females.(Kuhle et al, 2004; Stein et al, 2004).

The relatively higher incidence in neonates as compared to older children may be due to higher hematocrit, and the greater lability of the hemostatic system in neonates due to the generally decreased levels of both coagulation factors and their inhibitors in this age group, except factor VIII (FVIII) and von Willebrand factor (VWF) which are normal or even elevated.(Monagle et al, 2006) In adolescents the incidence equals that of young adults, probably due to the hormonal status, the use of contraceptives or pregnancy in young women, obesity and smoking.(Stein et al, 2004).

Clearly, these epidemiological data have to be considered when assessing the individual absolute thrombotic risk of children with thrombophilia.

3.2 Diagnosis

3.2.1 Clinical presentation

Pain, swelling and discoloration of extremities are acute symptoms of deep vein thrombosis (DVT). Vena cava inferior thrombosis manifests with prominent cutaneous veins and possibly liver or renal dysfunction depending on the site and extension of the thrombus. Superior vena cava thrombosis leads to cyanosis and swelling of the head and upper thorax with prominent collateral veins and may finally result in acute cardiac failure. Portal vein thrombosis, in most cases due to central catheters, and renal vein thrombosis with hematuria as a frequent sign may result in functional impairment or even failure of liver and renal function, respectively. Acute chest pain and dyspnea could suggest pulmonary embolism. Acute headache, visual impairment, cerebral convulsions and signs of venous congestion may indicate sinus venous thrombosis. Signs and symptoms of central venous catheter (CVC)-associated DVT are loss of CVC patency, the need for local thrombolytic therapy or CVC replacement, CVC-related sepsis, or prominent collateral circulation over chest, neck and head.

Childhood arterial ischemic stroke (AIS) manifests in neonates preferentially with seizures and abnormalities of muscle tone, whereas in elder children hemiparesis is the most frequent neurologic sign.(Steinlin et al, 2005) Acquired or inherited severe deficiencies of protein S and protein C are disorders involving both the microcirculation and arterial vessels and may manifest with characteristic symptoms such as deep skin necrosis (purpura fulminans), blindness due to retinal vessel occlusion and arterial embolism followed by necrosis of distal extremities or whole limbs. Thrombotic thrombocytopenic purpura (TTP), a severe microangiopathic disorder is characterized by nonimmunologic hemolytic anemia and thrombocytopenia, neurologic symptoms, and renal, pulmonary and cardial involvement.

3.2.2 Laboratory parameters

Every thrombotic event initiates a particular response to re-establish the balance of the hemostatic system, e.g., by fibrinolysis. Subsequently markers of fibrinolysis such as D-dimers can be detected in the circulation. The specificity of these markers is low; however, the negative predictive value of the D-dimer test to correctly exclude DVT is as high as 89% in adult patients with likely DVT compared to 99% in patients who were categorized as unlikely to have DVT.(Wells et al, 2003) In a study on the outcome of TE in children, elevated D-dimer and/or FVIII:C were found in only 67% of the patients; however, elevation of these markers at diagnosis and during follow-up are significantly correlated with persistence or recurrence of TE and/or a post-thrombotic syndrome. (Goldenberg et al, 2004)

3.2.3 Imaging

Color Doppler ultrasound, conventional and MRI angiography, lineograms and echocardiography are the diagnostic means of imaging the occlusion of vessels. Pulmonary embolism of proximal pulmonary arteries can be visualized by echocardiography and by CT scan; however, the specificity and sensitivity are low in detecting more distal clots. In such cases ventilation and perfusion scintigraphies are the recommended techniques for children.(Babyn et al, 2005) Transcranial Doppler ultrasound is used to assess the risk of stroke in patients with sickle cell disease. All techniques can be regarded as equally specific, sensitive and precise; their application, however, differs with respect to the region of interest, age and therapeutic options. **Table 3** lists the different techniques with respect to their application.

Method	**Indication**	**Limitations**
Lineograms	CVC related thrombosis	Only clots at the tip of the CVC and the distal adjacent vessel wall
Color Doppler ultrasound	DVT, SVT*	Exception: subclavian vein, use venography
Bilateral venography	DVT, SVT	Exception: jugular vein, use color Doppler ultrasound conventional or MRI
Echocardiography	CVC-related thrombosis, intracardial thrombus, pulmonary embolism	Distal clots in PE
Scintigraphy	Pulmonary embolism	–
Abbreviations: CVC, central venous catheter, DVT, deep vein thrombosis, SVT, Sinus venous thrombosis		
* in young infants through the patent fontanella.		

Table 3. Imaging methods for Thromboembolism in neonates and children.

3.3 Prothrombotic risk factors

Assessment of prothrombotic risk factors is by no means suitable for diagnosing TE. It may possibly help to explain unusual manifestations of TE; however, the predictive power concerning outcome, thereby providing a basis for therapeutic and prophylactic decisions is still a matter of ongoing studies and debate. Interpretation of laboratory data is strongly age dependent since normal ranges may differ considerably between newborns, young children and adolescents.

3.3.1 Hereditary prothrombotic factors

The most important factors involved in the genetic predisposition to thrombophilia are the factors of the coagulation cascade and in particular their natural inhibitors. It is not clear if genetic defects of fibrinolysis also contribute to the hypercoagulable state. Certain metabolic defects also cause thrombophilia.

3.3.1.1 Coagulation factors

3.3.1.1.1 Fibrinogen (FI)

In addition to being the final substrate for thrombin, FI is also an acute-phase protein that may lead to acquired thrombophilia and may also contribute to the risk of arterial TE.(Rothwel et al, 2004) Genetic defects causing dysfibrinogenemia associated with thrombophilia are rare.

3.3.1.1.2 Prothrombin (FII)

Heterozygosity for the 20210A allele of the common FII polymorphism 20210G/A in the untranslated 3 region of the Prothrombin (FII) gene (Poort et al, 1996) is found at a prevalence of 2.7% in the normal Caucasian population (*n* = 11.932, cumulative data from several studies). This mutant correlates with slightly elevated FII levels, suggesting a quantitative contribution to thrombophilia, and is found at a frequency of 7.1% in unselected patients with thombosis (*n* = 2884, cumulative data from several studies). The derived relative risk for thrombosis is 2.6. FII 20210A also seems to play a role in childhood stroke. Published data, however, do not give a clear picture.(Nowak - Gottl et al, 1999; Kenet et al, 2000) At least, FII 201210A does not seem to be involved in re-infarction.(Kurnik et al, 2003).

3.3.1.1.3 Factor V (FV)

The FV mutation Arg506 to Gln506 (R506Q or FV Leiden) causes relative resistance against cleavage by the activated protein C (PC) complex.(Dahlbäck et al, 1993; Bertina et al, 1994) It has been identified as the most common significant genetic risk factor for thrombosis to date. The prevalence in the normal Caucasian population is on the average 5%, with prevalences in particular populations of up to 15%.(Zoller et al, 1996) The relative thrombotic risk for heterozygotes is 6- to 8-fold, whereas homozygotes carry an 80-fold relative risk. (Koster et al, 1993) In children with venous thrombosis, FV Leiden was identified in up to 30%(Aschka et al, 1996) In contrast to adults it may also play a role in childhood stroke. (Nowak - Gottl et al, 1999)

3.3.1.1.4 Factor VIII (FVIII)

Elevated FVIII seems to contribute to the risk of TE in children. Furthermore, persistence of elevated FVIII after TE may also predict an unfavorable prognosis (Goldenberg et al, 2004), see Laboratory parameters.

3.3.1.1.5 Von Willebrand factor

Due to its key position in platelet adhesion and aggregation under conditions of high shear forces, VWF plays a most important hemostatic role in arterial vessels and in the microcirculation.(Ruggeri, 2004) This suggests a significant contribution of VWF to arterial TE and to microangiopathies such as thrombotic thrombocytopenic purpura (TTP). An elevated level of VWF is an independent risk factor for myocardial infarction and stroke in adults.(Vischer, 2006) It has not yet been shown whether elevated VWF also plays a role in arterial thrombosis of childhood. In the neonate, supra large VWF multimers, which are the most active in primary hemostasis, are more abundant than later in life and correlate with a very effective platelet dependent function of VWF in newborns.(Rehak et al, 2004) It can be speculated if these large multimers contribute to the higher rate of stroke in the perinatal period, but respective data have not been reported yet. However, it is now clear that supra large VWF multimers are responsible for the life-threatening condition of TTP (Lammle et al, 2005).

3.3.1.2 Inhibitors of hemostasis

The hemostatic process is tightly regulated by specific inhibitors that act on coagulation factors and on the factors of primary hemostasis. Functionally most important are tissue factor pathway inhibitor, the PC system, antithrombin (AT) and the VWF cleaving protease ADAMTS13. Clinically, to date only the latter three are important. Involvement of the coagulation inhibitors AT, PC and Protein S (PS) is rare with a prevalence in unselected patients with thrombosis of 0.019 for AT, 0.037 for PC, and 0.023 for PS deficiency.(Pabinger & Schneider, 1996; Koster et al, 1995) Recently, severe deficiency of ADAMTS13 has been identified as the causative factor of the rare TTP in most TTP patients (Lammle et al, 2005).

3.3.1.2.1 Protein C system

The PC system comprises PC, PS and FV as co-factors. PC is activated to APC by thrombin, which changes its substrate specificity from FI to PC by being bound to thrombomodulin at the endothelial cell surface. APC cleaves and inactivates aFV and aFVIII at specific proteolytic sites, thereby regulating the formation of thrombin. Severe PC deficiency as well as severe PS deficiency correlates with purpura fulminans, a life-threatening thromboembolic disorder of the microcirculation and larger vessels. Heterozygous deficiency of either inhibitor correlates with venous TE. PC also binds plasminogen activator inhibitor 1 (PAI1) which then facilitates fibrinolysis. This dual function of PC suggests a central role in the regulation of thrombus formation.

3.3.1.2.2 Antithrombin

When bound to heparan sulfate on endothelial cells, AT inhibits thrombin but also aFXI, aFIX and aFX. Its action on thrombin is enhanced 1000-fold by heparin through an allosteric conformational change. In contrast, low-molecular-weight heparin makes AT more aFX specific. These effects are the basis for prophylactic or therapeutic anticoagulation by heparin. Even mild hereditary deficiency of AT function may correlate with thrombophilia with a penetrance higher than in PC and PS deficiency.

3.3.1.2.3 ADAMTS13

ADAMTS13 regulates the size of VWF multimers and thereby its functional activity in primary hemostasis. Its deficiency has clearly been assessed as playing the causative role in TTP.(Lammle et al, 2005) An acquired form, caused by autoantibodies against ADAMTS13, and an inherited form called Upshaw Schulman syndrome (USS) due to mutations in the gene, exist. Lack of the protease correlates with persistence of supra large VWF multimers and, on an adequate trigger (infection, stress, hypoxia), these large multimers will induce platelet adhesion and aggregation in the microcirculation with subsequent microangiopathy, finally resulting in organ failure and death in 80% of cases when untreated. Thrombosis of larger venous and arterial vessels has also been observed. In childhood, TTP is rare and seems more often inherited.(Schneppenhim et al, 2004) Oligo-symptomatic courses have been observed, however, their long-term prognosis is not clear. In addition to the obvious causative role of severe ADAMTS13 deficiency in TTP, the impact of milder ADAMTS13 deficiency as thrombophilic factor has not been assessed yet, but is subject of ongoing studies. ADAMTS13 has been identified as a potent antithrombotic in an animal model, (Chauhan et al, 2006) which may be of future therapeutic interest.

3.3.1.3 Metabolic conditions

3.3.1.3.1 MTHFR polymorphism 677C/T

The rare condition of classical homocystinuria is most often caused by a deficiency of either cystathionine-ß-synthetase or 5-methyltetrahydrofolate-homocysteine-methyltransferase and correlates with frequent TE due to severe homocysteinemia causing endothelial cell damage. The activity of 5-methyl tetrahydrofolate-homocysteine-methyltransferase in turn depends on the availability of 5-methyl-tetrahydrofolate, regulated by 5, 10-methyl tetrahydrofolate-reductase (MTHFR). A common thermolabile MTHFR-variant (MTHFR, 677C>T) correlates with a slightly elevated level of homocysteine. Although repeatedly claimed in many studies, this variant does not seem to be an independent risk factor for TE.

3.3.1.3.2 Lipoprotein (a)

Lipoprotein (a) is considered a significant venous and arterial risk factor for TE in children.(Nowak - Gottl et al, 1999; Nowak - Gottl et al, 1999) However, other reports could not confirm these findings.(Revel - Vilk et al, 2003) Levels of Lp(a), though genetically determined, vary considerably among different populations. Lp(a) has structural homology to plasminogen, suggesting a possible competitive mechanism of Lp(a) in fibrinolysis. However, the lack of correlation between severe plasminogen deficiency and TE speaks against this hypothesis.

3.3.2 Acquired prothombotic risk factors

3.3.2.1 Central venous catheters

CVCs have become critically important as medical and supportive management of various diseases and have greatly improved quality of life. They bear two serious complications: thrombotic occlusion and CVC-associated DVT as well as systemic infections. CVCs seem to be the most important risk factor for DVT. The range of reported CVC-related DVT ranges from 1% to nearly 70%, reflecting the problem of different definitions, diagnostic methods and alertness.(Mitchell et al, 2003; Male et al, 2003) However, the estimated contribution of CVCs to all thromboembolic events in newborns is as high as 90% and over 50% in older children.(Parasuraman & Goldhaber, 2006) There are only a few controlled studies on the prevalence of CVC-related DVT and infection rate as well as the efficacy of antithrombotic measures to prevent catheter occlusion and infection.

3.3.2.2 Childhood cancer

TE is a well known complication in adult patients with cancer. With the exception of acute lymphoblastic leukemia (ALL), the knowledge about TE in childhood cancer is still limited. ALL has the highest rate of TE in childhood that is not necessarily related to the use of a CVC. In contrast, brain tumors have a rather low incidence of thrombosis with or without CVC.(Tabori et al, 2006) An overall estimation looks at a risk of up to 16%.

TE in cancer is the result of complex interactions of a variety of factors such as the malignancy itself, chemotherapy and its side effects including infections or dehydration, CVCs, the unbalanced hemostatic system with predominant hypercoagulability as well as possible hereditary thrombophilia. The impact of the different types of childhood malignancy on the hemostatic system is still not well understood. Most reports are regarding ALL and show the highest risk for TE under ALL/non-Hodgkin lymphoma (NHL) treatment is during induction and re-induction therapy that contains L-asparaginase, the most common site being the upper deep venous system and the cerebral veins.

3.3.2.3 Thrombosis and antiphospholipid syndrome (APS)

APS is an antibody-mediated thrombophilic state characterized by specific clinical manifestations of venous, arterial or small vessel TE at any site as well as the presence of antiphospholipid antibodies (APA) in the blood. In addition to DVT, acute ischemic stroke or transient ischemic attack are characteristic. APS is often associated with a number of autoimmune disorders.(Miyakis et al, 2006) APS in women causes adverse pregnancy outcome including unexplained still birth or prematurity because of severe placental insufficiency (multiple infarction) or severe (pre)eclampsia. APS is classified as primary and secondary; the clinical picture, however, is the same. Patients with no underlying disease are diagnosed as primary APS. Secondary APS refers to patients with underlying autoimmune (mainly rheumatologic) disorders as well as viral and bacterial infections or cancer.

All proposed pathophysiological mechanisms share the binding of the APA to anionic protein-phospholipid-complexes, leading to activation of endothelial cells, platelets and prothrombin, interference with natural inhibitory pathways and fibrinolysis, and disruption of the binding of annexin V to phospholipids coating the vascular system.(Levine et al, 2002; Rand, 2003) There are clinical/laboratory diagnostic and therapeutic criteria for adults (Miyakis et al, 2006) that do not apply equally for children. There have been recent reports on gene expression profiles to identify subtle distinctions in order to define the clinical relevance of different APA.(Ortel, 2006; Ortel, 2006) Apart from DVT as the most frequent clinical symptom in children along with the presence of LAC and high risk of recurrence without adequate long-term anticoagulation, there is a subgroup of children presenting with perinatal stroke and no risk of recurrence independent of secondary antithrombotic prophylaxis.(Kenet, 2006)This underlines the discordance to adults and the need for diagnostic and therapeutic guidelines to be defined for pediatric patients.

APA along with decreased activity of various coagulation factors, mainly F XII, are found in about 50% of otherwise healthy children with multiple viral infections, screened for prolonged a PTT preceding tonsillectomy or adenotomy.42-44 APA in this context are in association to the repeated infections and do not appear to be clinically relevant, carry no risk for bleeding or TE, and hence do not influence perioperative management. They usually disappear after tonsillectomy and/or with decreasing frequency of infectious episodes. In contrast, life-threatening TE including purpura fulminans may occur with varicella, which have been shown to have a increased prevalence of APA and associated PS deficiency.(Manco - Johnson, 1998) Bleeding is rare and responds to corticosteroids.

3.3.2.4 Heparin - induced thrombocytopenia type 2 (HIT)

The overall incidence of HIT type 2 is estimated around 1% of patients hospitalized in pediatric intensive care units.(Klenner et al, 2004; Newall et a, 2003) Most often it is observed in neonates and infants after cardiac surgery and in adolescents treated with unfractionated heparin (UFH) for venous thrombosis. HIT-associated TE is mainly venous but arterial events may occur.

3.3.2.5 Other acquired prothrombotic conditions

Perinatal asphyxia, systemic infections/sepsis/DIC, congenital heart disease (CHD) and hypovolemia are the main risk factors in neonates, the latter particularly prone to arterial events in association with CHD and/or arterial catheters frequently used in an intensive care setting.47 There are additional factors in older children: trauma, major surgery, immobilization, estrogen containing contraceptives in adolescent girls, corticosteroid therapy, nephrotic syndrome, hemolytic uremic syndrome, inflammatory bowel disease, and rheumatic and other chronic disorders. To date, it remains an individual decision if and which antithrombotic prophylaxis should be offered considering additional and individual risk factors.

3.4 Therapy and prophylaxis

Irrespective of an underlying disease, every thromboembolic manifestation should be treated, aiming at the complete recanalization of the occluded vessel and stopping the thrombotic process. In the vast majority of cases thrombosis will resolve under heparin given for 5–14 days. Other therapy options with a higher risk such as thrombolytic therapy or surgical embolectomy should be limited for patients with extensive thrombosis and/or threatened organ function. As LMWH show considerable advantages over UFH for therapeutic as well as prophylactic purposes, the following recommendations are in favor of LMWH. Yet evidence shows no difference in the antithrombotic efficacy. For detailed recommendations refer to **Table 4** and reference (Monagle et al, 2004).

UFH i.v.	**Neonates < 5kg**	**Children > 5kg**	**Target aPTT at 4h**
loading dose	1 x 75 U/kg/10 min	1 x 75 U/kg/10 min	
maintenance	25–30 U/kg/h	20 U/kg/h	60–85 sec.
LMWH s.c.	**Neonates < 5kg**	**Children > 5kg**	**Target anti-FXa at 4 h**
initial treatment dose			
Enoxaparin*	1 x 2.0 mg/kg/d	1 x 1.5 mg/kg/d	0.4–0.8 U/mL
Dalteparin	1 x 200 U/kg/d	1 x 150 U/kg/d	0.4–0.8 U/mL
Reviparin	2 x 150 U/kg/d	2 x 100 U/kg/d	0.5–1.0 U/mL
initial prophylactic dose			
Enoxaparin*	1 x 1.5 mg/kg/d	1 x 1.0 mg/kg/d	< 0.4 U/mL
Dalteparin	1 x 100 U/kg/d	1 x 50 U/kg/d	< 0.4 U/mL
Reviparin	2 x 50 U/kg/d	2 x 30 U/kg/d	< 0.5 U/mL

* 1 mg Enoxaparin = 110 anti-FXa units

For UFH: aPTT 4 hours after loading dose and 4 hours after each dosage adjustment, at least once daily; keep AT level within normal range; daily blood count (platelets!). For LMWH: anti-FX activity 4 hours after injection

Table 4. Recommended dosing of UFH and LMWH in neonates and children.

Recommendations

In children with VTE (CVL and non-CVL related): first TE for children:

In children with thrombosis, we recommend anticoagulant therapy with either UFH or LMWH (Grade 1B).

Remark: Dosing of IV UFH should prolong the aPTT to a range that corresponds to an anti-FXa level of 0.35 to 0.7 U/mL, whereas LMWH should achieve an anti-FXa level of 0.5 to 1.0 U/mL 4 h after an injection for twice-daily dosing.

We recommend initial treatment with UFH or LMWH for at least 5 to 10 days (Grade 1B). For patients in whom clinicians will subsequently prescribe VKAs, we recommend beginning oral therapy as early as day 1 and discontinuing UFH/LMWH on day 6 or later than day 6 if the INR has not exceeded 2.0 (Grade 1B). After the initial 5- to 10-day treatment period, we suggest LMWH rather than VKA therapy if therapeutic levels are difficult to maintain on VKA therapy or if VKA therapy is challenging for the child and family (Grade 2C).

We suggest children with idiopathic TE receive anticoagulant therapy for at least 6 months, using VKAs to achieve a target INR of (INR range, 2.0 to 3.0) or alternatively usingLMWH to maintain an anti-FXa level of 0.5 to 1.0 U/mL (Grade 2C).

Recurrent Idiopathic TE for Children

Recommendations

For children with recurrent idiopathic thrombosis, we recommend indefinite treatment with VKAs to achieve a target INR of 2.5 (INR range, 2.0 -3.0) [Grade 1A].

Remark: For some patients, long-term LMWH may be preferable; however, there are little or no data about the safety of long-term LMWH in children.

Recurrent Secondary TE for Children

Recommendations

For children with recurrent secondary TE with an existing reversible risk factor for thrombosis, we suggest anticoagulation until the removal of the precipitating factor but for a minimum of 3 months (Grade 2C). In addition, with specific respect to the managementof CVL-related thrombosis: 1.2.8. If a CVL is no longer required, or is nonfunctioning, we recommend it be removed (Grade 1B). We suggest at least 3 to 5 days of anticoagulation therapy prior to its removal (Grade 2C). If CVL access is required and the CVL is still functioning, we suggest that the CVL remain *in situ* and the patient be anticoagulated (Grade 2C).

For children with a first CVL-related DVT, we suggest initial management as for secondary TE as previously described. We suggest, after the initial 3 months of therapy, that prophylactic doses of VKAs (INR range, 1.5–1.9) or LMWH (anti-FXa level range, 0.1 to 0.3) be given until the CVL is removed (Grade 2C). If recurrent thrombosis occurs while the patient is receiving prophylactic therapy, we suggest continuing therapeutic doses until the CVL is removed but at least for a minimum of 3 months (Grade 2C).

Use of Thrombolysis in Pediatric Patients With DVT.

Recommendations

In children with DVT, we suggest that thrombolysis therapy not be used routinely (Grade 2C). If thrombolysis is used, in the presence of physiologic or pathologic deficiencies of plasminogen, we suggest supplementation with plasminogen (Grade 2C).

Thrombectomy and IVC Filter Use in Pediatric Patients With DVT.

Recommendations

If life-threatening VTE is present, we suggest thrombectomy (Grade 2C).

We suggest, following thrombectomy, anticoagulant therapy be initiated to prevent thrombus reaccumulation (Grade 2C).

In children _ 10 kg body weight with lower-extremity DVT and a contraindication to anticoagulation, we suggest placement of a temporary IVC filter (Grade 2C).

We suggest temporary IVC filters should be removed as soon as possible if thrombosis is not present in the basket of the filter and when the risk of anticoagulation decreases (Grade 2C).

In children who receive an IVC filter, we recommend appropriate anticoagulation for DVT (see 1.2) as soon as the contraindication to anticoagulation is resolved (Grade 1B).

Pediatric Cancer Patients With DVT

Use of Anticoagulants as Therapeutic Agents

Recommendations

In children with cancer, we suggest management of VTE follow the general recommendations for management of DVT in children.

We suggest the use of LMWH in the treatment of VTE for a minimum of 3 months until the precipitating factor has resolved (eg, use of asparaginase) [Grade 2C].

Remark: The presence of cancer, and the need for surgery, chemotherapy or other treatments may modify the risk/benefit ratio for treatment of DVT, and clinicians should consider these factors on an individual basis.

Use of Anticoagulant as Thromboprophylaxis

Recommendations

We suggest clinicians not use primary antithrombotic prophylaxis in children with cancer and central VADs (Grade 2C).

3.4.1 Commonly used anticoagulants

3.4.1.1 Unfractionated heparin

The following disadvantages should be considered: the need for venous access for therapy and monitoring, age-dependent unpredictable pharmacokinetics; normal AT levels required; monitoring by a PTT prone to pre-analytic errors; risk for bleeding; risk for HIT. Intravenous UFH should only be given in the initial phase of antithrombotic therapy and then switched to LMWH.

3.4.1.2 Low - molecular - weight heparin

Advantages are easy subcutaneous administration once daily without need of venous access, predictable pharmacokinetics, minimal monitoring, minimized bleeding complications, reduced risk of HIT. Infants < 5 kg required about 50% higher doses than older children to reach equivalent anti-FXa levels.(Sutor et al, 2004) As a general guideline we recommend LMWH with therapeutic anti-Xa levels for 4-6 weeks, followed by prophylactic dosage up to 6 months. For the treatment duration of different sites, types and age groups refer to references (Monagle et al, 2004; Andrew et al, 2000).

3.4.1.3 Thrombolytic agents

The agent of choice is rt-PA. Streptokinase should not be used because of its allergic reactions. The use of urokinase at least in the USA is restricted for safety concerns. rt-PA may be indicated if thrombosis is extensive or organ/life threatening. The established contraindications in adults apply for children as well but should be considered relative.53 Therapeutic recommendations are listed in **Table 5.**

Contraindications			
Strong	within 10 days after hemorrhage or major surgery		
	within 7 days after severe asphyxia		
	within 3 days after invasive procedure		
Soft	within 48 hours after cerebral convulsion		
	prematurity < 32 weeks of gestation		
	sepsis		
	active minor hemorrhage		
	refractory thrombcytopenia and hypofibrinogenemia		
Therapy	**Loading Dose**	**Maintenance**	**Monitoring**
rt-PA	0.1-0.2 mg/kg/10 min.	0.8-2.4 mg/kg/24 h	FI, platelets, D-dimers
UFH	none	5-10 U/kg/h	Apt
Indications: extensive and/or life/organ-threatening thrombosis. Contraindications: on an individual basis to be considered relative, not absolute; keep fibrinogen > 0.5 g/L and platelets > 50 g/L; increasing D-dimers indicate effective fibrinolysis; dose reduction or cessation of rt-PA if major bleeding occurs; minor bleeding (oozing from catheter puncture site or wound) treat with local pressure; optimal duration of rt-PA therapy uncertain, mostly up to 7 days, shorter/longer courses			

Table 5. Recommendations for systemic thrombolysis in neonates and children

3.4.1.4 Vitamin K antagonists

OAC	**Day 1**	**Day 2**	**From Day 3**	**Target INR**
Phenprocoumon	6 mg/m²	3 mg/m²	1-2 mg/m²	2.0-3.0
Warfarin	0.2 mg/kg	0.2 mg/kg	0.1-0.3 mg/kg	2.0-3.0
Reversal of oral anticoagulant therapy				
no bleeding, slow reversal	vitamin K 0.5-2.0 (-5.0) mg orally (s.c., i.v.)			
no bleeding, rapid reversal	vitamin K 0.5-2.0 (-5.0) mg s.c. or i.v.			
significant bleeding, not life threatening	vitamin K 0.5-2.0 (-5.0) mg s.c. or i.v. + FFP 20 mL/kg			
significant bleeding, life threatening	vitamin K 5 mg i.v. over 20 min. (risk of anaphylactic shock) + prothrombin concentrate (Prothomplex) 50 U/kg i.v.			
Coumarin therapy always to begin with concomitant heparin therapy (UFH or LMWH); to stop heparin, INR within therapeutic range for 2 days, concomitant medication at least 5 days; attention to multiple drug interactions				

Table 6. Recommended dosing of oral anticoagulants (OAC) in neonates and children.

Warfarin and phenprocoumon are usually administered for oral anticoagulation and inhibit g-carboxylation of vitamin K-dependent proteins. Considerable variation due to nutrition, co-medication, intercurrent illness and difficult monitoring requires close supervision and dose adjustment. We administer vitamin K antagonists in cases of prophylaxis exceeding 6 months (**Table 6**).

3.4.1.5 Infusion of deficient inhibitors of hemostasis

In cases of thrombosis with hereditary or acquired deficiencies of coagulation inhibitors, replacement therapy may be an option. Concentrates of AT and PC are commercially available and are life saving in conditions of purpura fulminans due to inhibitor deficiency. PC concentrate also proved to be effective in heterozygous or acquired PC deficiency. Fresh frozen plasma is the only but effective option of treating patients with purpura fulminans or hereditary TTP due to PS or ADAMTS13 deficiency, respectively.

3.4.2 New anticoagulants

The limitations of the traditional anticoagulants are particularly obvious in pediatrics; hence, the promotion of the new drugs already approved in adults urgent. Yet there is but individual experience in children with the following substances: the pentasaccharides fondaparinux and idraparinux, and the direct thrombin inhibitors hirudin, bivalirudin, argatroban; ximelagatran has been withdrawn from the market because of hepatic toxicity.(Balsa, 2005; Kuhle et al, 2006).

3.4.3 Special conditions

3.4.3.1 Prophylaxis of CVC occlusion

3.4.3.1.1 UFH

Prophylactic UFH seems to significantly decrease CVC-related DVT as well as bacterial colonization of the catheter.(Hentschen & Sutor, 2002) Heparin-bonded catheters do not reduce clot formation and bacterial colonization beyond 24 hours after CVC insertion.

3.4.3.1.2 Thrombolytic agents (urokinase, rt - PA)

Thrombolytic therapy is widely and safely used for the management of occluded catheters. There are only a few studies using thrombolytic agents prophylactically in order to reduce catheter infections and occlusions. Some studies show a substantial benefit of thrombolytic agents over UFH or no prophylaxis.(Hentschen & Sutor, 2002) whereas others get contradictory results.(Aquino et al, 2002; Solomon et al, 2000)

3.4.3.1.3 LMWH

Prophylactic use of LMWH has been efficient and safe in the treatment and prevention of DVT in children with cancer.(Elhasid et al, 2001; Massicotte et al, 2003; Tabori et al, 2006) However, LMWH to maintain CVC-patency and prevent CVC-related DVT has to remain an individual decision. For the recommended dosage see **Table 4**.

3.4.3.1.4 Oral anticoagulation with vitamin K - antagomist

There are no data for children on using low-dose oral anticoagulation to prevent CVC-associated DVT and to maintain catheter patency. Considering the heterogeneous pediatric population requiring a CVC with respect to age, thrombogenic risk profile, underlying disease, intensity and duration of treatment, the use of vitamin K-antagonists must remain a decision on a strictly individual base.

3.4.3.2 Management of Thrombosis in children with cancer

The main challenge is to keep the balance of benefit and risk of an antithrombotic treatment, as most children are being treated with chemotherapy with intermittent thrombocytopenia and an unbalanced hemostatic system, both of which lead to potential bleeding complications. It is therefore strongly recommended not to use antithrombotic agents with potentially serious side effects such as thrombolytic agents, UFH or vitamin K antagonists.

Recommendations

In children with cancer, we suggest management of VTE follow the general recommendations for management of DVT in children.

We suggest the use of LMWH in the treatment of VTE for a minimum of 3 months until the precipitating factor has resolved (*eg*, use of asparaginase) [Grade 2C].

Remark: The presence of cancer, and the need for surgery, chemotherapy or other treatments may modify the risk/benefit ratio for treatment of DVT, and clinicians should consider these factors on an individual basis.

3.4.3.3 Prophylaxis of TE in children with cancer

Since a high percentage of TE seems to be directly CVC-related, it is of primary importance to maintain its patency. Though there is a lack of clear evidence based indications the following situations for primary prophylaxis may be individually considered: 1) children with hereditary thrombophilia under intensive chemotherapy, 2) adolescents in the presence of additional risk factors such as major surgery or immobilization, 3) patients with prior TE in their history and 4) children with tumors compressing large vessels. Because ALL carries the highest risk for TE an efficient prophylaxis would be of major importance. To date there are no controlled trials that allow the extrapolation of prophylactic strategies. The German BFM-Study Group is conducting the first randomized interventional trial comparing three different antithrombotic strategies during ALL-induction therapy (Thrombotect). This ongoing trial is expected to provide the basis for risk adapted prophylaxis guidelines.

3.4.3.4 Antithrombotic therapy for APS

Long-term prognosis depends on the risk of recurrent TE, which seems to be the highest within 6 months of discontinuation of anticoagulation.64 Duration and intensity of therapy are still controversial, at least for subgroups. After the first DVT, secondary prophylaxis for 12 months is indicated. Lifelong anticoagulation is to be considered after a very serious first event and recurrent TE with persistence of APA. After arterial TE the optimal secondary prophylaxis remains controversial.64,65 In children consideration should be given to performing and/or extending first/second line antithrombotic treatment on an individual basis, depending on the presence of underlying disorders.

Recommendations

For children with VTE, in the setting of APLA (*Antiphospholipid Antibodies*), we suggest management as per general recommendations for VTE management in children.

Remark: Depending on the age of the patient, it may be more appropriate to follow adult guidelines for management of VTE in the setting of APLA.

3.4.3.5 Treatment - related indications for Thrombophilia Screening

It makes a difference if children are diagnosed and treated as study patients or if they are individually seen. In the latter case, laboratory work-up of thrombosis in childhood should pertain to the following basic questions: i) is there a specific therapy and ii) what are the consequences of a particular finding concerning future management and counseling of the patient and the family? (Sutor, 2003) Keeping this in mind, the necessary investigations are only a few (see **Table 7**) which is at odds with the current recommendations published by the Subcommittee on Perinatal/Pediatric Hemostasis of the Scientific and Standardization Committee (SSC) of the International Society on Thrombosis and Hemostasis (ISTH). (Manco - Johnson et al, 2002) However, since there is no consensus on management guidelines yet, laboratory testing may also vary between different institutions. It is well accepted that the coagulation inhibitors AT, PC and PS should be part of the diagnostic program. Though rare, their deficiencies can be compensated for by commercially available concentrates (AT, PC) and by fresh frozen plasma (PS). In cases of TE accompanied by hemolytic anemia and thrombocytopenia, Upshaw Schulman syndrome should be suspected and ADAMTS13 activity should be determined, since fresh-frozen plasma (FFP) is a life-saving replacement therapy in this condition and plasma exchange is the method of choice in the acquired form. Fasting homocysteine may be determined, since its elevation can be treated by folic acid substitution. However, two recent studies on lowering homocysteine by folate administration in patients with vascular disease did not show a reduction of re-infarction or stroke in adults.(Lonn et al, 2006; Ho et al, 2006) HIT type 2 should be ruled out in patients with thrombosis who show a drop of the platelet count under heparin administration. APA should be determined, since the respective patients require a longer lasting prophylaxis against a relapse. There is no specific treatment for patients with Factor V Leiden or PT G20210A. Although these established hereditary risk factors are the most common, therapeutic and prophylactic measures are not necessarily different for children with or without these risk factors. Indeed, many studies on adults and a few on children have shown that these factors have only minor or even no impact on re-TE in unselected patients with or without these risk factors.(Kurnik et al, 2003; Ho et al, 2006)

1	**2**	**3**
Antithrombin	APC resistance (FV Leiden)	PAI-1 polymorphism
Protein C	Prothrombin G20210A	Plasminogen
Protein S	Lipoprotein (a)	Heparin-cofactor II
Antiphospholipid-Ab	Dysfibrinogenemia	FIX
Homocysteine	FVIII	FXI
HIT Type 2	D-Dimer	FXIII
ADAMTS13		VWF
Column 1: factors of therapeutic and/or prognostic relevance; column 2: established risk factors with possible therapeutic and prognostic relevance for the individual patient; column 3: potential thrombophilic factors. Their therapeutic and prognostic relevance for the individual patient is doubtful. Laboratory tests for HIT type 2 and ADAMTS13 are only indicated when additional data suggest their involvement (see text).		

Table 7. List of relevant, established and potential thrombophilic factors

As some studies have suggested, combined thrombophilic factors may enhance the risk of thrombosis. However, the risk of a second event in unselected patients does not seem to be high enough to justify more intense and prolonged anticoagulation, compared to patients without these risk factors. Deviations from this "minimalistic" diagnostic approach may be indicated with respect to the individual case and to the particular institutional management guidelines. Many other factors are part of diagnostic programs, although their contribution to the thrombotic risk seems to be very low or even absent.

4. Acknowledgment

We are grateful to Mrs. Nathaly Zegarra Falen for their support the preparation of this chapter.

5. References

Abbott K et al Early renal insufficiency and late venous thromboembolism after renal transplantation in the United States. *Am J Kidney Dis* 2004 Jan; 43(1): 120-130

Adams M, Irish A, Watts G, Oostryck R and Dogra G. Hypercoagulability in chronic kidney disease is associated with coagulation activation but not endothelial function. *Thromb.Res.* 2008;123(2):374-380

Ageno W, Squizzato A, Garcia D, Imberti D. Epidemiology and risk factors of venous thromboembolism *Sem Thromb Haemost 2006;32(7):651-658*

Albisetti M, Schmugge M, Haas R, et al. Arterial thromboembolic complications in critically ill children. *J Crit Care.* 2005;20:296–300.

Allen R, Michie C, Murie J, Morris P Deep Vein Thrombosis After Renal Transplantation *Surg Gynecol Obstet* 1987;164: 137-42

Andrew M, Monagle P, Brooker L (Eds.) Thromboembolic Complications during Infancy and Childhood. B.C. Decker Inc., Hamilton, London: 2000

Ansell J, Hirsh J, Hylek E. et al. Pharmacology and management of the vitamin K antagonists : American College of Chest Physicians evidence-based clinical practice guidelines(8th ed). *Chest* 2008; 133:160S-198S.

Aquino VM, Sandler ES, Mustafa MM, Steele JW, Buchanan GR. A prospective double-blind randomized trial of urokinase flushes to prevent bacteremia resulting from luminal colonization of subcutaneous central venous catheters. *J Pediatr Hematol Oncol.* 2002; 24:710–713.

Arpino PA, Hallisey RK. Effect of renal function on the pharmacodynamics of. *Ann Pharmacother.* 2004;38:25–29

Aschka I, Aumann V, Bergmann F, et al. Prevalence of factor V Leiden in children with thromboembolism. *Eur J Pediatr.* 1996; 155:1009–1014.

Babyn PS, Gahunia HK, Massicotte P. Pulmonary thromboembolism in children. *Pediatr Radiol.* 2005;35: 258–274.

Bakhtawar K, Mahmoodi B et al High absolute risks and predictors of Venous and Arterial Thrmoboembolic Events in patients with Nephrotic Syndrome *Circulation* 2008 Jan 15;117(2):224-30

Balsa V. New Anticoagulants: A Pediatric Perspective. Pedaitr Blood Cancer. 2005;45:741–752

Bauer KA, Homering M, Berkowitz SD. Effects of age, weight, gener and renal function in a pooled analysis of four phase III studies of rivaroxaban for prevention of venous thromboembolism after major orthopedic surgery. *Blood (ASH Annual Meeting Abstracts)*. 2008;112:166-167. Abstract 436.

Beardsley D, Venous thromboembolism in the neonatal period. *Semin Perinatol* 2007;31:250-253

Berggwist D, Bergenta S, Bornmyr S, Husberg B, Konrad P, Liunger H Deep vein thrombosis after renal transplantation: A prospective analysis of frecuency and risk factors *Eur Surg Res* 1985; 17(2):69-74

Bertina RM, Koeleman BP, Koster T, et al. Mutation in blood coagulation factor V associated with resistance to activated protein C. Nature. 1994;369

Bonaa KH, Njolstad I, Ueland PM, et al; NORVIT Trial Investigators. Homocysteine lowering and cardiovascular events after acute myocardial infarction. N Engl J Med. 2006;354:1578–1588.

Chalmers EA. Epidemiology of venous thromboembolism in neonates and children. *Thromb Res* 2006;118:3-12

Chalmers EA. Perinatal stroke—risk factors and management. Br J Haematol. 2005;130:333–343.

Chauhan AK, Motto DG, Lamb CB, et al. Systemic antithrombotic effects of ADAMTS13. J Exp Med. 2006;203:767–776

Coush J, Selvin E, Stevens LA, et al. Prevalence of chronic kidney disease in the United States. *J Am Med Assoc* 2007; 298:2038-2047

Crowther M, Kelton J Congenital thrombofilia status associated with venous thrombosis a qualitative overview and proposed classification system *Ann Intern Med* 2003; 138:128-134

Dager W, Kiser T . Systemic Anticoagulation Considerations in Chronic Kidney Disease *Adv Chronic Kidney Dis* 2010;17(5):420-427

Dager WE, Dougherty JA, Nguyen PH, et al. Heparin-induced thrombocytopenia: Treatment options and special considerations. *Pharmacotherapy*. 2007;27:564–587

Dager WE. Initiating warfarin therapy *Ann Pharmacother*. 2003;37:905-908

Dahl OE, Kurth AA, Rosencher N, et al. Dabigatran etexilate150 mg once daily for the prevention of venous thromboembolism after total knee or hip replacement surgery in the elderly and those with moderate renal impairment. *J Thromb Haemost*. 2009;7(suppl 2):695-696.

Dahlbäck B, Carlsson M, Svensson PJ. Familial thrombophilia due to a previously unrecognized mechanism characterized by poor anticoagulant response to activated protein C: prediction of a cofactor to activated protein C. Proc Natl Acad Sci U S A. 1993;90:1004–1008.

Dillon PW, Jones GR, Bagnall-Reeb HA, Buckley JD, Wiener ES, Haase GM; Children's Oncology Group. Prophylactic urokinase in the management of long-term venous access devices in children: a Children's Oncology Group study. J Clin Oncol. 2004;22:2718–2723.

Elhasid R, Lanir N, Sharon R, Weyl Ben Arush M, Levin C, Postovsky S, Ben Barak A, Brenner B. Prophylactic therapy with enoxaparin during L-asparaginase treatment in children with acute lymphoblastic leukemia. Blood Coagul Fibrinolysis. 2001:12:367–370.

Follea G, Laville M, Pozet N. Pharmacokinetics studies of standard heparin and low molecular weight heparin in patients with chronic renal failure. *Hemostasis* 1986;16:147-51

Folsom A, Lutsey P, el al Atherosclerosis Risk in Communities Study *Nephrol Dial Trasplant* 2010 Oct 25(10):3256-3301

Frost C, Yu Z, Nepal S, Mosqueda-Garcia R, Shenker A. Apixaban, an oral direct Factor Xa inhibitor: single-dose safety, pharmacokinetics and pharmacodynamics in healthy volunteers. *J Thromb Haemost.* 2007;5(suppl 1).

Frost C, Yu Z, Moore K, et al. Apixaban, an oral direct factor Xa inhibitor: multiple-dose safety, pharmacokinetics, and pharmacodynamics in healthy subjects. *J Thromb Haemost.* 2007;5

Giroud M, Lemesle M, Gouyon JB, et al. Cerebrovascular disease in children under 16 years of age in the city of Dijon, France: a study of incidence and clinical features from 1985 to 1993. J Clin Epidemiol. 1995;48:1343–1348.

Goldenberg NA, Knapp-Clevenger MSN, Manco-Johnson MJ. Elevated Factor VIII and D-dimer levels as predictors of poor outcomes of thrombosis in children. N Engl J Med. 2004;351:1081–1088.

Grand'Maison A, Charest A, Geerts W. Anticoagulant Use in Patients with Chronic Renal Impairment. *Am J Cardiovasc Drugs* 2005;5(5)291-305

Haidl H, Cimenti C, Leschnik B, Zach D, Muntean W. Age-dependency of thrombin generation measured by means of calibrated automated thrombography (CAT). Thromb Haemost. 2006;95:772–775.

Harder S, Renal profiles of *anticoagulants J Clin Pharmacol.* Published on line 24 May 2011 http://jcp.sagepub.com/content/early/2011/05/24/0091270011409231

Heller C, Schobess R, Kurnik K, et al. 2000. Abdominal venous thrombosis in neonates and infants: role of prothrombotic risk factors - a multicentre case-control study. For the Childhood Thrombophilia Study Group. *Br J Haematol,* 111:534–9.

Hentschel R, Sutor A. Katheterthrombosen im Kindesalter und ihre Prävention. Hämostaseologie. 2002;22:167–173.

Hirsh J, Bauer K, Donati MB, el al Parenteral anticoagulants :American College of Chest Physicians evidence-based clinical practice guidelines(8th ed*) Chest 2008;* 133:141S-159S

Ho WK, Hankey GJ, Quinlan DJ, Eikelboom JW. Risk of recurrent venous thromboembolism in patients with common thrombophilia: a systematic review. Arch Intern Med. 2006;166:729–736.

Hursting MJ, Murray PT. Argatroban anticoagulation in renal dysfunction: A literature analysis. *Nephron.* 2008; 109:c80–c94

Ignjatovic V, Summerhayes R, Than J, et al. 2006. Therapeutic range for unfractionated heparin therapy: age-related differences in response in children. *J Thromb Haemost,* 4:2280–2.

Ignjatovic V, Summerhayes R, Gan A, et al. 2007. Monitoring unfractionated Heparin (UFH) therapy: which anti-factor Xa assay is appropriate? *Thromb Res*, 120:347–51.

Irish A. Hypercoagulability in renal Transplant Recipients : Identifying patients at risk of renal allograft thrombosis and evaluating strategies for prevention *Am J Card Drugs* 2004:4(3):130-140

Jackson C, Graves M, Patterson A el al. Relationship between platelet aggregation, thromboxane synthesis and albumin concentration in nephrotic syndrome. *Br J Haematol* 1982;52:69-77.

Kayali F,Najjar F, Aswed F, Natta F and Sein P Venous Thromboembolism in patients hospitalized with Nephrotic Syndrome *Am J Med* 2008 March ; 121(3):226

Kearon C, Kahn S, Agnelli G et al. Antithrombotic Therapy for Venous Thromboembolic Disease American College of Chest Physicians Evidence-Based Clinical Practice Guidelines (8th Edition) *Chest* 2008; 133:454S–545S

Kearon C, Ginsberg JS, Julian JA el al. Comparision of fixed-dose weight-adjusted unfractionated heparin and low- molecular- weight heparin for acute treatment of venous thromboembolism. *JAMA* 2006;1296;935-942

Kenet G. Perinatal/Pediatric Haemostasis Subcommittee of the SSC of the ISTH, Minutes and Annual Reports 2006, 52nd Annual SSC meeting of the ISTH, Oslo 2006.

Kenet G, Sadetzki S, Murad H, et al. Factor V Leiden and antiphospholipid antibodies are significant risk factors for ischemic stroke in children. Stroke. 2000;31:1283–1288.

Keush G. Thrombotic complications in the nephritic syndrome. *Schweiz Med Wochenschr* 1989 Aug 8;119(31-32):1080-5

Keller C, Katz R, Cushman M , Fried L. Association of kidney function with inflammatory and procoagulant markers in a diverse cohort: a cross-sectional analysis from the Multi-Ethnic Study of Aterosclerosis(MESA) *BMC Nephrol* 2008;9:9.

Kiser TH, Burch JC, Klem PM, et al. Safety, efficacy, and dosing requirements of bivalirudin in patients with heparin-induced thrombocytopenia. *Pharmacotherapy.* 2008;28:1115-1124

Koster T, Rosendaal FR, Briet E, et al. Protein C deficiency in a controlled series of unselected outpatients: an infrequent but clear risk factor for venous thrombosis (Leiden Thrombophilia Study) Blood. 1995;85:2756–2761.

Koster T, Rosendaal FR, de Ronde H, Briet E, Vandenbroucke JP, Bertina RM. Venous thrombosis due to poor anticoagulant response to activated protein C: Leiden Thrombophilia Study. Lancet. 1993;342:1503–1506.

Klenner A, Lubenow N, Raschke R, et al. Heparin-induced thrombocytopenia in children: 12 new cases and review of the literature. Thromb Haemost. 2004;91:719–723

Kubitza D, Becka M, Mueck W, et al. Effects of renal impairment on the pharmacokinetics, pharmacodynamics and safety of rivaroxaban—an oral, direct Factor Xa inhibitor. *Br J Clin Pharmacol.* 2010;70:703-712.

Kuhle S, Massicotte P, Chan A, et al. Systemic thromboembolism in children: Data from the 1-800-NO-CLOTS Consultation Service. Thromb Haemost. 2004;92:722–728.

Kuhle S, Lau A, Bajzar L, et al. Comparison of the anticoagulant effect of a direct thrombin inhibitor and a low molecular weight heparin in an acquired antithrombin deficiency in children with acute lamphoblastic leukaemia treated with L-asparaginase: an in vitro study. Br J Haematol. 2006;134:526–531

Kurnik K, Kosch A, Strater R, Schobess R, Heller C, Nowak-Göttl U. Recurrent thromboembolism in infants and children suffering from symptomic neonatal arterial stroke: a prospective follow-up study. Stroke. 2003;34:2887–2892.

Lammle B, Kremer Hovinga JA, Alberio L. Thrombotic thrombocytopenic purpura. J Thromb Haemost. 2005;3:1663–1675.

Levine JS, Branch DW, Rauch J. The antiphospholipid syndrome. N Engl J Med. 2002;346:752–763.

Lim W, Crowther MA, Eikelboom JW. Management of antiphospholipid antibody syndrome: a systematic review. JAMA. 2006;295:1050–1057.

Lim W, Dentali F, Eikelboom JW, et al Meta-analysis:low-molecular-weight heparin and bleeding in patients with severe renal insufficiency. *Ann Intern med*,2006;144:673-684

Limdi Na, Beasley TM, Baird MF et al. Kidney function influences warfarin responsiveness and hemorrhagic complications. *J Am Soc Nephrolo*. 2009; 20: 912-921

Lisman T, De Groot G, Meijers J, Rosendaal F. Reduced plasma fibrinolytic potential is a risk factor for venous thrombosis *Blood* 2005 ;105(3): 1102-1105

Lobo BL, Use of newer anticoagulants in patients with chronic kidney disease *Am J Health Syst Pharm* 2007,Oct 1;64(19):2017-26.

Lonn E, Yusuf S, Arnold MJ, et al; Heart Outcomes Prevention Evaluation (HOPE) 2 Investigators. Homocysteine lowering with folic acid and B vitamins in vascular disease. N Engl J Med. 2006;354:1567–1577.

Lynch J, Hirtz D, deVeber G, Nelson K. Report of the National Institute of Neurological Disorders and Stroke Workshop on perinatal and childhood stroke. Pediatrics. 2002;109:116–123.

Manco-Johnson MJ. Antiphospholipid antibodies in children. Semin Thromb Hemost. 1998;24:591–598.

Manco-Johnson MJ, Grabowski EF, Hellgreen M, et al. Laboratory testing for thrombophilia in pediatric patients. On behalf of the Subcommittee for Perinatal and Pediatric Thrombosis of the Scientific and Standardization Committee of the International Society of Thrombosis and Haemostasis (ISTH). Thromb Haemost. 2002;88:155–156.

Male C, Chait P, Andrew M, Hanna K, Julian J, Mitchell L; PARKAA Investigators. Central venous line-related thrombosis in children: association with central venous line location and insertion technique. Blood. 2003;101:4273–4278.

Massicotte P, Julian JA, Gent M, Shields K, Marzinotto V, Szechtman B, Chan AK, Andrew M; PROTEKT Study Group. An open-label randomized controlled trial of low molecular weight heparin for the prevention of central venous line-related thrombotic complications in children: the PROTEKT trial. Thromb Res. 2003;109:101–108.

Mitchell LG, Andrew M, Hanna K, et al; Prophylactic Antithrombin Replacement in Kids with Acute Lymphoblastic Leukemia Treated with Asparaginase Group (PARKAA). A prospective cohort study determining the prevalence of thrombotic events in children with acute lymphoblastic leukemia and a central venous line who are treated with L-asparaginase: results of the Prophylactic Antithrombin Replacement in Kids with Acute Lymphoblastic Leukemia Treated with Asparaginase (PARKAA) Study. Cancer. 2003;97:508–516.

Miyakis S, Lockshin MD, Atsumi T, et al. International consensus statement on an update of the classification criteria for definite antiphospholipid syndrome (APS). J Thromb Haemost. 2006;4:295–306.

Mitchell LG, Andrew M, Hanna K, et al ; Prophylactic Antithrombin Replacement in kids with Acute Lymphoblactic Leukemia Treated with Asparaginase Group (PARKAAA). A prospective cohort Study determining the prevalence of thrombotic events in children with acute lymphoblastic leukemia and central venous line who are treated with L - asparaginase: results of the Prophylactic Antithrombin Replacement in kids with Acute Lymphoblastic Leukemia Treated with Asparaginase (PARKAAA) Study. Cáncer. 2003; 97: 508 - 516.

Monagle P, Chalmers E, Chan A, deVeber G, Kirkham F, Massicotte P & Michelson A. (2008) Antithrombotic therapy in neonates and children: American College of Chest Physicuans evidence-based clinical practice guidelines (8th edition*), chest, pp* Vol.133 (june 2008),*.pp. 887S-968S.*

Monagle P & Andrew M.(2003). Chapter: Development hemostasis: relevance to newborns and infants, In: Hematology of infancy and childhood, Nathan D, Orkin S, Ginsburg D & Look A, pp. (121-168), Saunders.

Mizumoto H, Maihara T, Hiejima E, et al. Transient antiphospholipid antibodies associated with acute infections in children: a report of three cases and a review of the literature. Eur J Pediatr. 2006;165:484–488.

Monagle P, Barnes C, Ignjatovic V, et al. Developmental haemostasis: Impact for clinical haemostasis laboratories. Thromb Haemost. 2006;95:362–372.

Monagle P, Chan AK, Massicotte P, et al. Antithrombotic therapy in children. Chest. 2004;126:645S–687S.

Newall F, Barnes C, Ignjatovic V, et al. Heparin-induced thrombocytopenia in children. J Paediatr Child Health. 2003;39:289–92.

Nowak-Gottl U, Junker R, Hartmeier M, et al. Increased lipoprotein(a) is an important risk factor for venous thromboembolism in childhood. Circulation. 1999;100:743–748.

Nowak-Gottl U, von Kries R, Gobel U. Neonatal symptomatic thromboembolism in Germany: two year survey. *Arch Dis Child Fetal Neonatal* Ed 1997;76(3):F163- 67.

Nowak-Göttl U, Strater R, Heinecke A, et al. Lipoprotein (a) and genetic polymorphisms of clotting factor V, prothrombin, and methylenetetrahydrofolate reductase are risk factors of spontaneous ischemic stroke in childhood. Blood. 1999;94:3678–3682.

Ocak G, Verduijn M et al *Chronic kidney disease stages 1-3 increase the risk of venous thrombosis. J ThrombHaemost* 200 Nov;8(11): 2428-35

Ortel TL. The antiphospholipid syndrome: what are we really measuring? How do we measure it? And how do we treat it? J Thromb Thrombolysis. 2006;21:79–83.

Ortel TL. The Lupus anticoagulant Subcommittee of the SSC of the ISTH, Minutes and Annual Reports 2006, 52nd Annual SSC meeting of the ISTH, Oslo 2006.

Ortel TL. Thrombosis and the antiphospholipid syndrome. Hematology (Am Soc Hematol Educ Program). 2005;462–468.

Pabinger I, Schneider B. Thrombotic risk in hereditary antithrombin III, protein C, or protein S deficiency. A cooperative, retrospective study. Gesellschaft fur Thrombose- und Hamostaseforschung (GTH) Study Group on Natural Inhibitors. Arterioscler Thromb Vasc Biol. 1996;16:742–748.

Parasuraman S, Goldhaber SZ. Venous thromboembolism in children. Circulation. 2006;113:e12–e16.

Poli D, Zanazzi H, Antonucci E, Bertoni E , Salvadoti M, Abbate R, Prisco D Renal trasplant recipients are at high risk for both symptomatic and asymptomatic deep vein thrombosis *J Thromb Haemost* 2006 May;4(5):988-92

Poort SR, Rosendaal FR, Reitsma PH, Bertina RM. A common genetic variation in the 3'-untranslated region of the prothrombin gene is associated with elevated plasma prothrombin levels and an increase in venous thrombosis. Blood. 1996;88:3698–3703.

Rand JH. The antiphospholipid syndrome. Annu Rev Med. 2003;54:409–424.

Rehak T, Cvirn G, Gallistl S, et al. Increased shear stress-and ristocetin-induced binding of von Willebrand factor to platelets in cord compared with adult plasma. Thromb Haemost. 2004;92:682–687.

Revel-Vilk S, Chan A, Bauman M, Massicotte P. Prothrombotic conditions in an unselected cohort of children with venous thromboembolic disease. J Thromb Haemost. 2003;1:915–921.

Revel-Vilk S, Chan A, Bauman M, Massicotte P.Prothrombotic conditions in an unselected cohort of children with venous thromboembolic disease. *J Thromb Haemost* 2003; 1:915–21.

Rosendaal F. Venous thromboembolism : a multicausal disease. *Lancet* 1999;353:1167-1173

Rothwell PM, Howard SC, Power DA, et al. Fibrinogen concentration and risk of ischemic stroke and acute coronary events in 5113 patients with transient ischemic attack and minor ischemic stroke. Stroke. 2004;35:2300–2305.

Roy M, Turner Gomes S, Gill G. Incidence and diagnosis of neonatal thrombosis associated with umbilical venous catheters. *Thromb Haemost* 1997; 78:724

Ruggeri ZM. Platelet and von Willebrand factor interactions at the vessel wall. Hamostaseologie. 2004;24:1–11.

Siøland J et al. Fibrin clot structure in patients with end-stage renal disease *Thromb Haemost* 2007 Aug;98(2):339-345

Shantsila E, Lip GY. Apixaban, an oral, direct inhibitor of activated Factor Xa. *Curr Opin Investig Drugs*. 2008;9:1020-1033.

Schneppenheim R, Budde U, Hassenpflug W, Obser T. Severe ADAMTS-13 deficiency in childhood.

Stangier J. Clinical pharmacokinetics and pharmacodynamics of the oral direct thrombin inhibitor dabigatran etexilate. *Clin Pharmacokinet*. 2008;47:285-295.

Schmidt B, Andrew M. Neonatal thrombosis: report of a prospective Canadian and international registry. *Pediatrics* 1995;96(5 Pt 1):939- 43.

Semin Hematol. 2004;41:83–89.

Solomon B, Moore J, Arthur C, Prince HM. Lack of efficacy of twice-weekly urokinase in the prevention of complications associated with Hickman catheters: a multicentre randomised comparison of urokinase versus heparin. Eur J Cancer. 200;37:2379–2384.

Stein PD, Kayali F, Olson RE. Incidence of venous thromboembolism in infants and children: data from the national hospital discharge survey. J Pediatr 2004;145:563–565.

Steinlin M, Pfister I, Pavlovic J, et al; The Swiss Societies of Paediatric Neurology and Neonatology. The first three years of the Swiss Neuropaediatric Stroke Registry (SNPSR): a population-based study of incidence, symptoms and risk factors. Neuropediatrics. 2005;36:90–97.

Sutor AH. Screening children with thrombosis for thrombophilic proteins. Cui bono? J Thromb Haemost. 2003;1:886–888.

Sutor AH, Chan AK, Massicotte P. Low-molecular-weight heparin in pediatric patients. Semin Thromb Hemost. 2004;30 Suppl 1:31–39.

Tabori U, Beni-Adani L, Dvir R, et al. Risk of venous thromboembolism in pediatric patients with brain tumors. Pediatr Blood Cancer. 2004;43:633–636. Wiernikowski JT, Athale UH. Thromboembolic complications in children with cancer. Thromb Res. 2006;118:137–152.

Turebylu R, Salis R, Erbe R, Martin D, Lakshminrusimha S, Ryan RM. Genetic prothrombotic mutations are common in neonates but are not associated with umbilical catheter-associated thrombosis. *J Perinatol* 2007; 27:490–5.

Tveit D, Hypolite I et al. Chronic dialysis patients have high risk for pulmonary embolism. *Am J Kidney Dis* 2002 May;39(5):1011-1017.

Undas A, Kolarz N, Koped G, Traczl W Altered fibrin clot properties in patients on long term haemodyalisis:relation to cardiovascular mortality. *Neph Dial Transplant* 2007 ;23(6):2010-2015.

van Ommen CH, Heijboer H, Buller HR, Hirasing RA, Heijmans HS, Peters M. Venous thromboembolism in childhood:a prospective two-year registry in The Netherlands.*J Pediatr* 2001;139(5):676- 81

Vaziri N, Branson H, Ness R Changes of coagulation factors IX,VIII,VII,X and V in Nephrotic Syndrome *Am J Med Sci* 1980;280:167-171

Vaziri N, Paule P,Toohey J el al. Acquired deficiency and urinary excretion of antithrombin III in nephrotic syndrome *Arch Intern Med* 1984;144:1802-1803

Veldman A, Nold M, Michel-Behnke I. Thrombosis in the critically ill neonate: incidence,diagnosis and management. *Vascular Health and Risk Management* 2008:4(6) 1337–1348

Vischer UM. von Willebrand factor, endothelial dysfunction, and cardiovascular disease. J Thromb Haemost. 2006;4:1186–1193.

Wattanakit K, Cushman M, Stehman b, Heeckbert S,Falsom A. Chronic kidney disease increases risk for venous thromboembolism. *J Am Soc Nephrol* 2008;19:135-140

Wells PS, Anderson DR, Rodger M, et al. Evalutation of D-dimer in the diagnosis of suspected deep-vein thrombosis. N Engl J Med. 2003;349:1227–1235.

Zoller B, Norlund L, Leksell H, et al. High prevalence of the FVR506Q mutation causing APC resistance in a region of southern Sweden with a high incidence of venous thrombosis. Thromb Res. 1996;83:475–477.

4

Venous Thromboembolism in Cancer Patients

Galilah F. Zaher[1] and Mohamed A. Abdelaal[2]
[1]*Haematology – Faculty of Medicine, King Abdulaziz University, Jeddah,*
[2]*Haematologist Princess Noorah Oncology Center, Head of King Abdullah International Medical Research Center, King Abdulaziz Medical City, Jeddah, Saudi Arabia*

1. Introduction

Venous Thromboembolism (VTE) is a major complication of cancer and is one of the leading causes of death in patients with cancer. The risk for VTE in this group of patients is increased several folds in hospitalized cancer patient and in those on active therapy. The short and long term consequences of VTE diagnosis in cancer patients are many including increased in mortality rate, bleeding while on therapy for VTE. It has, therefore, become important to identify the risk factors for cancer-associated VTE, develop guidelines for prevention strategies for high-risk patients as well as management of VTE when it complicates the course of cancer disease or its treatment with chemotherapy immunomodulatory agents, antiangiogenesis or hormonal therapy. Proper understanding of the epidemiology and pathophysiology of VTE and its risk factors in cancer patients is central to adequate prevention and management of this serious complication in cancer patients.

2. The epidemiology and pathophysiology of venous thrombosis in cancer patients

2.1 Cancer cells and the haemostatic mechanisms

The haemostatic system is a complex, multifaceted mechanism that participates in maintaining the integrity of the vascular system and fluidity of blood. In coordination with the mechanisms of inflammation and repair, the haemostatic mechanism produces a coordinated response. Haemostatic systems are normally quiescent and are only activated after injury and results in the production of a platelet plug, fibrin-based clot, deposition of white cells at the site of injury, and activation of inflammatory and repair processes.

Tumor cells can activate blood coagulation through multiple mechanisms, including (a) production of procoagulant, fibrinolytic, and proaggregating activities; (b) release of proinflammatory and proangiogenic cytokines and (c) direct interaction with host vascular and blood cells through adhesion molecules.

Miller et al (1) studied the link between the haemostatic systems and cancer where the authors evaluated haemostatic status every year for 4 years in a population of approximately 3000 middle-aged men without cancer. Among patients with the activation of the haemostatic system (defined as persistent elevation of fibrinopeptide A and prothrombin fragment 1+2 levels), total mortality was significantly higher in participants with persistent activation (17.1/1000 person-years) than in patients without activation (9.7/1000 person-years; p=0.015). This difference was attributed to an increased incidence of death from cancers (11.3/1000 vs. 5.1/1000 person-years).

The majority of patients with cancer has increased levels of procoagualnt factors V, VIII, IX, and XI, as well as increased levels of markers of coagulation activation (e.g., thrombin-antithrombin, prothrombin fragment 1+2, fibrinopeptide and D-dimer (2). In addition, patients with some disseminated malignancies seem to have a deficient activity of von Willebrand's factor-cleaving protease (ADAMTS-13), resulting in unusually large von Willebrand factor multimers leading to platelet thrombosis (3).

Many tumors have been shown to activate blood coagulation through an abnormal expression of high levels of the procoagulant molecule tissue factor (TF). In normal vascular cells, expression of TF is not expressed, except when induced by inflammatory cytokines such as interleukin 1β and tumor necrosis factor α (TNF-α) or by bacterial lipopolysaccharides. In tumor cells, TF is expressed and causes activation of the extrinsic pathway. In the elegant study conducted by Kakkar et al (4) plasma levels of TF, factor VIIa, factor XIIa, the thrombin-antithrombin complex, and prothrombin fragments were elevated in patients with cancer compared with healthy controls. Tissue factor and factor VIIa levels were both significantly higher, suggesting significant activation of the extrinsic pathway. On the other hand, levels of factor XIIa were only marginally elevated, indicating that the intrinsic pathway is not involved to a significant degree in the hypercoagulable state seen in patients with cancer (5).

Tumor cells express cancer procoagulant, a cysteine protease expressed only on malignant tissues. Cancer procoagulant directly activates factor X in the common pathway independent of factor VII (6). The activity of this protease seems to be driven by the stage of cancer. The onset of cancer is usually associated with high levels of protease slowly declines thereafter (7), partially explaining the tendency of thromboembolic events to occur during the first three month following the diagnosis of cancer.

In addition to the expression of TF and cancer procoagulant, tumor cells enhance coagulation in patients with cancer by expressing proteins that regulate the fibrinolytic system, including plasminogen activators, plasminogen activator inhibitors 1 and 2, and plasminogen-activator receptor, leading to an imbalance of fibrinolytic mechanism (8) Tumor cells may elicit platelet activation and aggregation through direct cell-cell interactions or through the release of soluble mediators, including ADP, thrombin, and other proteases. Furthermore, expression of certain cytokines by tumor cells, including TNF-α and interleukin 1β, induces expression of TF on endothelial cells and simultaneously downregulates the expression of thrombomodulin, resulting in a prothrombotic state at the vascular wall.Multiple studies have provided considerable evidence for a bidirectional clinical association between VTE and cancer, in that cancer elicits expression of procoagulant activities, contributing to the prothrombotic state in these patients, and the procoagulant activities themselves seem to elicit cancer growth, proliferation, and metastasis. Fibrin and platelet deposition around solid tumor cells promotes angiogenesis through platelet-derived proangiogenic factors, and may seal immature tumor vasculature and provide a degree of protection to the cancer cells from the immune system. Fibrin has also been shown to increase expression of TF and induce expression of IL-8 and vascular endothelium growth factor (VEGF) and thereby, enhancing angiogenesis (9-10).

The TF–factor VIIa complex can signal through cleavage of protease-activated receptors, which, in turn, induce the mitogen-activated protein kinase (MAPK) signal transduction cascade (11). The MAPK pathway is involved in the induction of genes involved in angiogenesis, migration, and proliferation. In addition, phosphorylation of the cytoplasmic tail of the TF receptor has also been shown to indirectly activate transcription of VEGF, downregulate thrombospondin (an antiangiogenic protein), and induce cell migration. Expression of TF by malignant cells also seems to support metastatic process and is dependent on the formation of the TF-factor VIIa complex (11).

2.2 The incidence of venous thromboembolism in cancer patients

The first description of deep vein thrombosis (DVT) in patients with cancer was made by Bouillard in 1823(12) although this was popularly first credited to Armand Troussean, the French Physician, in 1865 (13-14). Since that time, hundreds of studies have provided solid data on the clinical association between VTE and cancer, and delineated the elevated risk for VTE particularly during the first few months following the diagnosis of cancer and in the presence of distant metastasis (15-18).

The incidence of DVT or PE in patients with cancer varies widely because of the heterogeneity of the patients' population and the difficulty of conducting large epidemiological studies. Based on a prospective medical database in the United States, the annual incidence of a first episode of DVT or PE in the general population is 0.1% (15), while the estimated annual incidence of VTE in the cancer population is 0.5%. (19-21) The prevalence of cancer-associated thrombosis may be underestimated by more than 10-fold as autopsy studies in cancer patients have demonstrated even higher rates of VTE (17-22). In a large population-based epidemiological study, approximately 20% of all new cases of VTE are associated with underlying cancer, whereas 26% of incident cases had idiopathic VTE (15).

The risk of VTE associated with different malignancies has more recently been quantified in NHL (23), colonic cancer (24) ovarian (25) lung (26) and breast cancer (27). It was generally thought that solid tumors, such as pancreatic, ovarian and brain cancer carry a much higher risk for VTE than haematological malignancies. However, recent studies suggest that the incidence of VTE in patients with haematological malignancies may be similar to that observed in patients with solid tumors (28). In a population based case-control study of patients with a first episode of VTE, Blom et al found that the odds ratio of developing VTE among patients with haematological malignancies was approximately 26 compared to the general population (18). Similar results were also reported by other authors (29-31).

Prospective studies has shown that VTE have inflicted a higher risk of several adverse complications on patients with cancer including recurrent VTE, bleeding complications while on anticoagulant treatment, increase in both short-term and long-term mortality (32-33) and increased mortality during first 3 month of therapy. The risk of VTE is markedly different for cancer patients throughout the course of the disease and this variable incidence of VTE comorbidity in cancer patients can be attributed to a combination risk factors related to the patient, the cancer itself and treatment (34).

2.3 Patient-related factors and risk of VTE

a. **Age:** Older age has been shown to be associated with VTE in hospitalized cancer patients, but not in ambulatory patients (35-37). The rate of VTE in patients older than 60 years of age undergoing surgery for various solid tumors was significantly higher than that in younger patients by multivariate analysis (OR 2.6) (36-38).

b. **Gender:** Among cancer patients, most studies have identified male gender as a significant predictor of VTE. (19-20) However, A recent pooled retrospective study of VTE rates in a large cohort of hospitalized cancer patients reported a higher rate in females (OR 1.1, $p < 0.0001$) (39)

c. **Race:** In the general population, the incidence of VTE varies by race. In the USA, it is highest among blacks and lowest among Asian-Pacific Islanders (40).

d. **Previous thrombotic episode:** Cancer patients with a past history of VTE have a 6–7 fold increased risk of developing VTE compared to those with no history of VTE (38).

e. **Obesity** has been confirmed to be an important risk factor in cancer-associated thrombosis. Body mass index ≥35 kg/m^2 was identified as one of five variables in a risk prediction model proposed by Khorana et al with an OR of 2.1 (38)

f. **Chronic co-morbid Medical Conditions:** The presence of chronic medical co-morbid conditions such as chronic renal disease, chronic liver disease, hypertension and chronic heart failure has a marked effect on the incidence of cancer-associated thrombosis and survival. The presence of three or more chronic medical conditions was the strongest risk factor for development of VTE among the patients with gliomas and ovarian cancer, and was the second strongest risk factor among patients with breast or colon cancer (39-40).

2.4 Cancer-related factors to incidence of VTE

a. **Tumor type:** certain tumors are strongly associated with VTE. In the retrospective cohort study of hospitalized cancer patients. Khorana et al (38), reported that sites of cancer with the highest proportion of patients with VTE were pancreas, brain and endometrial or cervical were 12.1%, 9.5% and 9%, respectively (California Cancer Registry). The incidence of VTE in pancreatic cancer patients is at least 10-fold higher than the rate in patients with prostate cancer. Histological subtype also predicts the increased risk of VTE in some types of malignancy. The incidence of VTE in patients with non-small cell lung cancer was 9.9% in patients with adenocarcinoma subtype versus 7.7% in patients with squamous cell carcinoma (HR 1.9, CI 1.7–2.1) (27, 26). Although mucin production was once proposed as the common feature and the thrombogenic mechanism amongst these mucin-producing tumors, the exact pathogenesis of the prothrombotic state of mucin is still not fully understood.

b. **Initial cancer stage:** Patients diagnosed with local-stage cancer, in general, have a very low incidence of VTE, whereas the incidence is much higher in patients diagnosed with metastatic disease at time of diagnosis (24-27).

c. **Biological aggressiveness of cancer:** The observed differences in the incidence of VTE between different cancer types correlate with the biological behavior of the cancer. A very strong correlation was found between the 1- year fatality rate and the 1-year cumulative incidence of VTE (41). In addition, presence of metastatic disease at the time of diagnosis is a strong independent risk factor for developing VTE within the first year of cancer diagnosis (42-43).

d. **Rate of metastatic spread:** The incidence of VTE has been reported to correlate with the rate of growth and spread of the cancer cells. Fast growing cancer such as colonic and ovarian, has been associated with a higher rate of VTE (24-25, 41-42) and patients with advanced and metastatic disease had a higher risk of VTE (OR 19.8, CI 2.6–149). The observed incidence of VTE in ovarian, colorectal, pancreatic, lung and breast cancer supports the finding that advanced stage increases the risk of cancer associated VTE (24-25, 44).

2.5 Cancer Treatment-related factors and risk of VTE

2.5.1

Chemotherapy is one of the most important treatment-related factors in the aetiology of cancer-associated VTE as cancer alone is associated with a four-fold risk of thrombosis, while chemotherapy increases the risk by six-fold (45-47)

Several different mechanisms have been reported to explain the prothrombotic states induced by chemotherapy including (a) damage to the vascular endothelium (48-49), (b) reduction of endogenous, physiological, anticoagulant factors (56-59), (c) increase of levels of procoagulants (54-57), (d) induction of tumor and endothelial level apoptosis and cytokine release that, in turn, lead to increased expression and hence activity of TF (56-57), (e) induction of platelet activation (58) and (f) direct induction of expression of monocyte-macrophages TF (59).

The following chemotherapeutic agents are associated with high risk for VTE:

- **Cisplatin based regimens**

Weiji et al (60), in a retrospective review of VTE in germ cell cancer patients treated with cisplatin and bleomycin-based chemotherapy reported an estimated risk of thrombosis of 8.4%. In a prospective study of VTE in non-small cell lung cancer patients treated with cisplatin and gemcitabine, Numico et al (61) reported VTE incidence of 17.6%.

The mechanisms by which cisplatin induces thrombosis is not well known but in vitro studies suggest increase in the level of TF (48), platelet activation (50) and increased levels of von Willebrand factor suggesting endothelial injury (58). The latter perhaps explain the cisplatin induced arterial thrombosis. Moore et al (62) conducted a large retrospective analysis to determine the incidence of venous and arterial thromboembolic events in patients treated with cisplatin-based chemotherapy and confirmed the unacceptable incidence of those events and recommend randomized studies to examine the question of prophylactic anticoagulation in patients with cancer treated with chemotherapy.

- **L-Asparaginase**

L-Asparaginase (ASNase) has been a mainstay in the treatment of paediatric patients with acute lymphoblastic leukemia since the 1960's and there are several reports of ASNase containing regimen used in the treatment of paediatric ALL achieving a higher survival rate than non-ASNase treatment regimens used for ALL in adults and adolescents (63-65).

L-Asparaginase converts L-Asparagine to L-aspartic acid and, thereby, reduces levels of L-Asparagine, an essential amino acid for protein synthesis and as a result, leukemic cell growth is inhibited. However, the production of multiple plasma proteins by the liver including haemostatic factors, is also reduced and hence causing marked disruption of the haemostatic mechanism: prolongation of PT and aPTT, reduced fibrinogen level, reduced levels of protein C and protein S, Antithrombin III (AT) , plasminogen, factor IX and factor XII. On the other hand, ASNase causes increased procoagulant factors V, VIII (54-56). In addition, to the profound effects of the drug on the pro- and anticoagulant molecules, ASNase has also been shown to increase levels of immunomodulin a marker of vascular injury (66).

The simultaneous effects of ASNase on both procoagulant and thrombolytic proteins increase the risk of both bleeding and thrombosis, the latter being the main challenge.

The incidence of ASNase - associated VTE complications is age-dependent, 3-5% in children (67, 31) whereas the incidence reported from Dana-Farber Cancer Institute (1991-2008) in adult patients (≥ 30 years) was 34% and 42% (68). Less intensive ASNase regimen in adult patients have reported lower rates of thrombotic complications (69). Limited reports and data on a small number of patients treated with pegASNase -related DVT may be less frequent than those treated with after E. Coli ASNase (70-74). In UKALL 2003, Children with DVT were routinely retreated with pegASNase and concurrent heparin prophylaxis without recurrence of thrombosis (75). The confounding factors for VTE during ASNase therapy are presence of indwelling catheter, oral contraception, prednisolone and inherited thrombophilia (76).

The majority of clinically important thrombotic events were those related to venous catheters and those in the central nervous system. The majority of catheter-associated thrombosis (CAT) are asymptomatic and the majority, in both children and adults, occur during induction (68).

In the randomized trial of native ASNase versus pegASNase (74), the incidence of cerebral venous sinus thrombosis (CVST) of 2-3% in children was reported. In children ≥ 10 years, initial WBC > 50×10^9 /L at diagnosis may predict higher risk for CVST (77). The GIMEMA study on adult ALL patients protocol, including E. Coli ASNase in the induction phase, CNS thrombotic events was 3% (77).

Prevention and Management of ASNase induced thrombosis

Primary Prevention: In children and adolescents prophylaxis is rarely undertaken and there has been few reports that the use of AT concentrate may decrease the incidence of thrombosis (78-79)

In a historically controlled study of adult patients, Mitchell et al (78) reported that the incidence of VTE was lower in a cohort of patients who received prophylactic AT concentrate but the study did not establish efficacy. A retrospective comparison of cohort of patients at two centers in Canada who had prophylaxis against CNS thrombosis with fresh frozen plasma and cryoprecipitate did not develop CVST (80).

Most paediatric oncology centers do not perform the coagulation screening tests or perform AT levels routinely. If prophylaxis is deemed appropriate for a particular patient, it is best applied during induction phase of therapy when the majority of VTE events take place.

For intracranial thrombohemorrhagic complications, the use of AT concentrates and/or cryoprecipitates to replace both AT and fibrinogen, respectively, is a reasonable approach. In case of unavailability of AT, fresh frozen plasma (FFP) at a dose of 20 ml/kg can raise the AT level by approximately 20%. However, FFP may also replenish asparagine and, thereby, counteract the anti-leukemic effect of ASNase. There is no clear indication from the literature about whether further administration of ASNase should be stopped in adults after a thrombotic event while on therapy. In children, ASNase is continued under cover of low-molecular-weight heparin. Patients with thrombotic events after ASNase have been successfully re-challenged with ASNase without recurrence of thrombosis (75). In the Dana-Farber Cancer Institute review (63) confirms that, after venous thromboembolic events, asparaginase can be restarted after demonstrating clot stabilization or improvement by imaging with close monitoring of anticoagulation. Therefore, a history of venous thromboernbolic events does not seem to adversely impact prognosis.

The expert panel, Wendy Stock et al (81) in their excellent article published in Leukemia and Lymphoma, 2011 detailed the management of ASNase associated VTE and put down the recommendation which is being adapted/summarized hereunder:

1. In adults, activated partial thromboplastin time (APTT), international normalized ratio (INR), AT, and fibrinogen levels should be measured prior to ASNase therapy for baseline assessment.
2. Between doses of native ASNase and for 1 week after pegASNase therapy, these tests, as well as factor Xa, should be serially monitored as clinically indicated.
3. AT concentrates and cryoprecipitate infusions should be considered for treatment of thrombohemorrhagic events due to AT and fibrinogen deficiency, respectively.
4. For non-urgent thrombohemorrhagic episodes, fresh frozen plasma should be avoided since it contains asparagine and may counteract the anti-leukemic effect of ASNase. However, careful follow up is advised for possible evolution of the thrombohemorrhagic event into a major one.
5. For a clinically significant DVT, the patient should be anticoagulated with or without AT supplementation, and whether or not it is associated with a central venous line.
6. Early diagnostic imaging, CT scan and or MRI should be performed in patients with a suspected CNS event related to ASNase therapy and urgent consultation of the neurologist/ neurosurgeon should be secured and documented.
7. For CNS thrombosis, the patient should be anticoagulated with or without AT supplementation after careful evaluation.
8. Anti-epileptic medications in patients with thrombohemorrhagic complications should be administered prophylactically or therapeutically as appropriate at the discretion of the neurologist.
9. ASNase is discontinued for all clinically significant bleeding or thrombosis and whether it is resumed depends on the nature and resolution of the thrombohemorrhagic event and outcome of discussion of the case at the tumor board.

5-Fluorouracil

This synthetic pyrimidine analogue is an important chemotherapeutic agent for treatment of various solid tumors. The incidence of VTE in patients treated for colorectal cancer with this drug has been reported at 15-17%. During 5-FU infusion, there is a reduction of protein C and an increase level of fibrinopeptide through the action of thrombin (83-84).

2.5.2 Angiogenic Inhibitors and immunomodulatory agents

a. Angiogenesis Inhibitors Associated with VTE:

Angiogenesis is a process involving the proliferation of new blood vessels and plays a central role in the growth and metastasis of cancer (85). The angiogenesis is driven mainly by the vascular endothelial growth factor (VEGF). The signaling pathway of VEGF has been a target of many angiogenesis inhibitors including bevacizumab, sorafenib and others (86-87). Bevacizumab (Avastin, Genentech Inc., South San Francisco California) is a recombinant humanized monoclonal neutralizing antibody against VEGF has shown efficacy in treatment of many solid tumors including colorectal cancer, non-small cell lung cancer and renal cell carcinoma.

Shobha R Nalluri et al (88) in their metanalysis of 15 randomized controlled trials (RCTs) demonstrated that bevacizumab is associated with significantly higher risk of VTE (RR, 1.33[95% CI 1.13-1.56]; $P<0.001$) in patients with a variety of metastatic solid tumors and this risk is observed for all grades of VTE.

The thrombogenic effect of bevacizumab may be related to (a) its exposure of the subendothelial procoagulant layer and inhibition of the VEGF induced endothelial cell regeneration (89), (b) reduction of production of nitric oxide and prostacyclin by bevacizumab (90), (c) release of procoagulant molecules from the tumor cells into the circulation (91) and (d) increasing the haematocrit and blood viscosity via over production of erythropoietin (92).

b. Thalidomide and its derivative Lenalidomide are immunomodulatory agents with antiangiogenic properties through blockade of basic fibroblastic growth factor and VEGF and are associated with increased risk of VTE in cancer patients. This topic has been well covered in chapter 5 of this book by Drs Gonzalez-Porras and Mateos.

2.5.3 Hemopoetic growth factors

Tumor hypoxia may contribute to the resistance of some tumors to both chemotherapy and radiation therapy (93-94). Many cancer patients are anemic. There are some data from the literature indicating that patients who received transfusions to maintain a higher hematocrit have improved outcomes with radiation therapy for cervical carcinoma. (95)

Studies on inducing and maintaining higher haemoglobin (Hb) levels in patients with malignant disease by administration of recombinant human erythropoietin (rHuEpo), the primary haematopoietic growth factor for erythropoiesis (96), have shown that rHuEpo is effective in increasing Hb levels in the majority of anaemic cancer patients (97-98) and that this increase is associated with an improvement in patient-reported quality of life. Because both fatigue and anemia are common complications of cancer, the use of rHuEpo in patients with cancer has increased significantly (99). Those studies typically have shown that a majority of patients will have an erythropoietic response to doses of rHuEpo between 150 IU/kg and 300 IU/kg given subcutaneously 3 times per week (98, 100).

Dusenbery et al (101) in a study of patients receiving rHuEpo along with chemotherapy and radiation therapy for cervical carcinoma, reported that 2 of 20 patients had DVT during therapy, and 2 other patients had DVT 9 days and 10 days after radiation therapy and rHuEpo were discontinued. Although it was a small sample, the rate of 20% in that study is similar to the rate found in by Ted Wun et al (102). The combination of chemotherapy and radiation may lead to a more vigorous inflammatory response that may predispose patients to thrombosis in the background of other predisposing factors.

In a recent Cochrane meta-analysis of 35 trials representing almost 7000 patients, epoetin or darbepoetin treatment was associated with a significantly increased risk for thromboembolic events (103).

Erythropoietin may contribute synergistically to thrombosis in cancer patients through several mechanisms. (a) Increasing red cell mass leading to increasing whole blood viscosity, (b) Erythropoietin therapy results in reticulocytosis, the metabolically active young red blood cells. Elegant studies have demonstrated that metabolically active red blood cells augment platelet reactivity in vitro (104-108) (c) rHuEpo is synergistic with the platelet growth factor, thrombopoietin, for platelet activation in vitro (109-110) at concentrations that can be achieved pharmacologically in vivo. (d) Erythropoietin has been associated with increased platelet reactivity and evidence of endothelial activation when administered to healthy male volunteers (111) (e) In vitro data have demonstrated receptor-mediated endothelial cell activation in response to rHuEpo and that extracellular matrix produced by the activated endothelial cells enhanced platelet aggregation and recent evidence suggests that platelet-red cell interactions can play a role in venous thrombosis (112).

The role of prophylactic myeloid growth factors: granulocyte colony stimulating factor (G-CSF) and granulocyte-macrophage colony stimulating factor (GM-CSF) in increasing risk of cancer-associated thrombosis is unclear (113-114).

2.5.4 Surgery

Is a well-known risk factor for development of VTE in patients without cancer. Underlying cancer increases the risk of surgery-related VTE by two-fold. Some studies have demonstrated that longer time in the operating room, longer time under anesthesia, and need for surgical re-exploration is associated with increased risk of VTE in cancer patients (37, 115-116). A study analyzing the effect of surgery in patients with glioma revealed that patients who underwent major neurosurgery or brain biopsy were 70% more likely to develop VTE within 3 months.

2.5.5 Indwelling central venous catheters (CVC)

The use of CVC has improved the management of patients with cancer as they simplified the administration of chemotherapy, parental nutrition, antibiotics and other supportive intravenous therapy. However, the CVCs are associated with complications including a significant risk of catheter-associated thrombosis (CAT). The risk of VTE associated with hospitalization has increased over the last decade a time associated with increased use of medical thromboprophylaxis. The incidence of symptomatic catheter-related DVT in adult cancer patients ranges from 0.3% to 28% while the rate of catheter-related DVT assessed by venography is 27–66% (117).

Some of the factors that may influence the risk of thrombosis of the indwelling central lines are (a) site of the catheter: left subclavian lines are at higher risk than the right (b) synthetic material: polyvinyl chloride or polyethylene lines are more thrombogenic than are polyurethane or siliconized lines (c) number of lumen: triple lumen catheters may be more thrombogenic than double lumen (d) nature of the infusate: infusion of total parenteral nutrition fluids through the line have been found to be more thrombogenic than the infusion of crystalloid fluids (e) the position of the tip of the catheter located in the superior vena cava has almost a three-fold higher risk for thrombosis than that located in the right atrium and (f) insertion attempts of ≥2 carries higher risk for catheter related thrombosis.

Patient with CAT may present with pain, swelling, paresthesia, and prominent veins throughout the arm or shoulder. However, many patients may be asymptomatic.

Contrast venography is the gold standard for evaluation of patients suspected to have the upper extremity thrombosis. However, the non-invasive serial compression ultrasound is the standard test for UEDVT evaluation and if this is negative in a patient with high-pretest probability of UEDVT then the more expensive and invasive ultrasonography is resolved to.

In some centers, Color Doppler duplex ultrasound may be the modality of choice for the diagnosis of symptomatic CVC-R of UEDVT and for screening of suspected asymptomatic thrombosis in specific clinical situations (118)

Prevention: Despite the strong association between the CVCs and UEDVT, anticoagulant prophylaxis is not recommended. Studies evaluating the use of 1-mg (low dose) warfarin gave conflicting results (119-121).

On the basis of the available data from contemporary trials, it is difficult to recommend routine antithrombotic prophylaxis in cancer patients with central venous catheters. Institutions are encouraged to assess their rates of catheter-associated thrombosis and develop a protocol on how the catheters are inserted and maintained. This will be a useful tool to control the rate of complications associated with CVCs. When symptomatic thrombosis occurs in association with a catheter, it definitely complicates the clinical care of the patient because of the need for anticoagulant therapy and because often the catheter has to be removed.

Management of Catheter Associated Thrombosis

Treatment: ACCP guidelines recommend treating UEDVT patient with UH or LMWH and warfarin (INR 2-3) for at least 3-months (122).

- **Right Atrial Thrombus**

a. **Surgical management**

These thrombi may impede atrial or ventricular inflow and cause sudden death. For a symptomatic patient with a large mobile thrombus, surgical thrombectomy is strongly recommended (123-124) and the catheter should also be explanted (125, 126, 127). Early involvement of the cardiologist, the cardiac surgeon and intensivist is advisable for coordinated optimum management.

b. Medical management

A completely dissolved right atrial thrombus case without side effects was reported by Adamovich et al in a neonate after 5 days' with infusion of urokinase and heparin (128). Cesaro et al reported on a successful pediatric case that was treated with recombinant tissue plasminogen activator (rt-PA) and heparin for 6 days without significant side effects (129). Korones et al favoured conservative management for small-sized thrombus with no intervention but close follow up for evidence of growth in size is warranted. However, for a moderate-sized thrombus there is a need for anticoagulation rather than surgical thrombectomy (123). If medical treatment fails then surgical thrombectomy should be resolved to. In adults, medical treatment has been tried in only a few reported cases because it is believed that, even though antithrombotic agents may stabilize or regress catheter-related RA thrombi, anticoagulated patients remain at risk of pulmonary embolism and need to have surgical thrombectomy eventually (130-132).

- **Central Venous Thrombosis**

a. Surgical management

The course of action for implantable venous access device (IVAD) after CVT is variable. Medical antithrombotic treatment was widely applied, but most of the devices were still explanted and some were removed before medical treatment is started (5,6) and some were explanted after fibrinolytic, antithrombotic or anticoagulant treatment failed (133-135). The reasons for explantation of IVAD are (a) prevention of thrombosis progression, especially in the case of SVC syndrome, (b) persistent pain, (c) combined with a documented infection and extravasation. However, Lokich et al (136) reported that the vascular occlusion rarely resolve after the explantation.

b. Medical management

For all CVT patients with or without IVAD explantation, antithrombotic treatment is necessary. Removal of the device should be decided by clinical necessity for venous access or by evidence of pulmonary embolism (134), especially in patients with very difficult venous access.

c. Unfractionated Heparin

Intravenous UFH is the initial treatment of choice for acute CVT. UFH can prevent clot propagation but does not dissolve it and, therefore, recanalization may not develop. UFH can be given by continuous intravenous infusion for 5–10 days, starting with a bolus of 5000 IU followed by 30,000–35,000 IU/day, with activated partial thromboplastin time of 1.5-2.5 times the control (137).

d. Low Molecular Weight Heparin

In view of the many advantages particularly the subcutaneous route q12 hours dosage, no need for laboratory and home treatment basis of the LMWH over the UFH, many experts favor its use for management of acute CVT

e. Fibrinolytic agents

Fibrinolytic agents, such as recombinant tissue plasminogen activator (rt-PA), streptokinase, and urokinase are usually effective for the lysis of fresh thrombi. Resolution of thrombi is more significant in acute occlusions than in CVT, which is always detected after a period of time i.e. chronic organized thrombosis. Although some studies mentioned their usage, antithrombotic agents are still the first choice (134,138).

- **Intraluminal thrombotic occlusion**

a. **Surgical management**

Surgical explantation of the device should be considered after fibrinolytics have failed or therapy has been terminated because of its minor severity and the high success rate of medical treatment (134,139-140).

b. **Medical treatment**

Fibrinolytic agents, such as rt-PA, urokinase and streptokinase, have been used in recent decades to lyse intraluminal thrombi, to restore device patency and to avoid catheter removal. Intraluminal installation of fibrinolytic agents is still considered the safest and most effective therapy for the treatment of IVAD intraluminal thrombotic occlusions. These agents are associated with some complications e.g. bleeding, hypersensitivity reactions, arrhythmias, hypotension, fever, nausea or vomiting and the attending physician is advised to make note of this at the time when a decision is made.

c. **Recombinant tissue-plasminogen activator (rt-PA)**

Alteplase is the most popular and effective rt-PA used in the treatment of thrombotic occlusions. It is a serine protease that activates plasminogen to plasmin in the cleavage of thrombus-bound fibrin. In adult patients, 2 mg alteplase in 2 mL sterile water may be injected into the occluded catheter. Restoration of function is assessed 30–120 minutes later and if function is not restored, a second attempt with the same dose is performed (141-142). In 64-86% of patients successful treatment was achieved after a single dose, and two doses achieved 81–94% success. In addition, alteplase has the advantages of a low incidence of allergic reactions (< 0.02%) and no documented reports of sustained antibody formation after administration (134). Although small dose alteplase is so far not commercially available, large dose alteplase can be split into unit doses and cryopreserved at -20°C for 30 days (141). Reconstruction to small dose aliquots makes this a cost-effective treatment without compromising safety and efficacy (141-142). However, the production of a single-dose rt-PA vial is still needed, not only for small institutions but also as a convenient, economically sound and safe agent for oncologic patients.

d. **Urokinase**

In 1999, the FDA reported on microorganism contamination of urokinase and issued a warning about variations in quality control during manufacture, recommending that urokinase be restricted to specific patients in whom the physician has judged urokinase to be critical to the clinical situation (143).

e. **Streptokinase**

Although streptokinase can resolve occlusions without hemorrhagic side effects or coagulation changes. Its use is fraud with some difficulties: allergic reactions and the induction of antibody formation, fever and shivering in 1–4% and anaphylactic reactions 0.1% of patients these risks/issues led to the restriction of its usage (141,144). The producers of streptokinase, AstraZeneca, released an Important Safety Information letter on streptokinase in December 1999 and warned that there is a risk of significant allergic reactions and that streptokinase is not indicated for restoration of IVAD patency (144).

2.5.6 Radiation

There are limited data on the effect of isolated radiation modality on risk of cancer-associated thrombosis. However, the combination of chemotherapy and radiation could lead to a more vigorous inflammatory response that may predispose patients to thrombosis in the setting of other predisposing factors. In a study of patients receiving rHuEpo along with chemotherapy and radiation therapy for cervical carcinoma, Dusenbery et al (101) reported that 2 of 20 patients had DVT during therapy, and 2 other patients had DVT 9 days and 10 days after radiation therapy and rHuEpo were discontinued. Although it was a small sample, the rate of 20% in that study is remarkably close to the rate found by other investigators. Large, randomized studies of combined chemotherapy and radiation therapy in patients with carcinoma of the cervix did not report on the rate of venous thrombosis (145-148).

2.5.7 Hormonal therapy: Tamoxifen and exemestane

Tamoxifen was discovered by pharmaceutical company Imperial Chemical Industries (now AstraZeneca) and is sold under the trade names Nolvadex, Istubal, and Valodex. However, the drug, even before its patent expiration, was and still widely referred to by its generic name "tamoxifen."

Tamoxifen binds to estrogen receptors but produces both estrogenic and antiestrogenic effects. It reduces circulating insulin-like growth factor-1, inhibits angiogenesis, and induces apoptosis (149)

Tamoxifen is highly beneficial as adjuvant therapy for breast cancer, and more recently, its effectiveness has been demonstrated for prevention of breast cancer in high-risk women. (150-151)

The most frequent side effect in patients treated with tamoxifen versus placebo was a doubling of the rate of DVT and PE: 118 versus 62 cases and a similar increase in superficial phlebitis (68 versus 30 cases) (152) A systematic review of adjuvant hormonal therapy for breast cancer estimated that women treated with 5 years of tamoxifen have a 1.5-7.1 fold increased risk of VTE compared to women treated with placebo or on observation only. (153)

As to the evaluation of women who are about to initiate tamoxifen to prevent the development of breast cancer, the question raised is cost: benefit ratio of tamoxifen therapy if the patient have risk factors for DVT or PE. On the basis of the solid data favoring tamoxifen, the prevention of breast cancer should take priority over the risk of venous thromboembolism. If the risk of developing DVT is high, it is reasonable to go for concomitant anticoagulation with Coumadin (INR 2-3) for the planned treatment period with tamoxifen.

However VTE risk may become less problematic in breast cancer patients as the third-generation oral aromatase inhibitors, such as the irreversible steroidal inactivator exemestane, are being used in place of tamoxifen for long-term prophylaxis after initial therapy of breast cancer. Exemestane is the generic name for the brand-name drug Aromasin and works by binding irreversibly to the body's aromastase enzyme, which is responsible for producing estrogen. Many breast cancer cells depend on estrogen to grow and multiply quickly. Once the aromatase inhibitor binds to the aromastase enzyme, the bound aromatase enzyme can no longer produce estrogen. This drug caused lack of estrogen "starves" estrogen- dependent breast cancer cells, preventing them from multiplying. Coombes et al, in a trial in which 4742 breast cancer patients were randomized to continue tamoxifen or to switch to exemestane. Those receiving exemestane experienced improvement in disease-free survival (154-155) The adjusted hazard ratio was 0.67 (95% CI 0.56 to 0.82, P<0.001) and the rate of thromboembolic events was almost halved in those receiving exemestane as compared with tamoxifen (1.3% versus 2.4%, p=0.007).

3. VTE and occult cancer

Thrombosis can be the first manifestation of malignancy. Patients who present with idiopathic or unprovoked DVT are more likely to be diagnosed with cancer during follow-up than patients with secondary DVT. In pooled analyses of cohort studies, the odds ratio for subsequent cancer in patients presenting with idiopathic VTE compared with patients with secondary VTE is 4.8 (156). About 10% of patients with idiopathic VTE were diagnosed with subsequent cancers over the next 5–10 years. More than 75% of these cases were reported within the first year after the diagnosis of DVT (157).

Prins et al studied (158) the incidence of newly diagnosed malignancy in patients with unexplained venous thromboembolism during the first year after a thromboembolic event in comparison to controls (odds ratio, 3.9-36). The authors used extensive screening with computed tomography, endoscopy and tumor markers and stated that they identify most of these undetected malignancies. However, the authors continued, approximately half of these can also be identified based on a simple clinical evaluation.

Monreal et al (159) reported on retrospective analysis of our 5-year experience with a series of 674 consecutive otherwise healthy patients, and a more restricted battery of diagnostic tests including: abdominal CT-scan; carcinoembryonic levels, and prostate-specific antigen levels. The authors reported that cancer was more commonly found in patients with idiopathic VTE: 13/105 patients (12%) versus 10/569 patients (2%); p <0.01; O.R.: 7.9 (95% CI: 3.14-20.09). During the same period of time they diagnosed VTE in 147 patients with previously known cancer. When overall considered, VTE was the first sign of malignancy in most patients with prostatic and pancreatic carcinoma. However, most patients with breast, lung, uterine and brain cancers developed VTE as a terminal event of the disease (159).

Piccioli et al (160) also concurred with Monreal et al (159) that the diagnosis of venous thrombosis although may help to uncover previously occult carcinoma by prompting a complete physical examination, chest roentgenography, and mammography, extensive cancer screening with computed tomography to neck, chest, abdomen and pelvis or magnetic resonance imaging has not been shown to be cost effective for patients with venous thrombosis.

In another publication, Piccioli et al (161) reported that patients with symptomatic idiopathic venous thromboembolism and apparently cancer-free have an approximate 10% incidence of subsequent cancer. In their study, apparently cancer-free patients with acute idiopathic venous thromboembolism were randomized to either the strategy of extensive screening for occult cancer or to no further testing. Patients had a 2-year follow-up period. Of the 201 patients, 99 were allocated to the extensive screening group and 102 to the control group. In 13 (13.1%) patients, the extensive screening identified occult cancer. In the extensive screening group, a single (1.0%) malignancy became apparent during follow-up, whereas in the control group a total of 10 (9.8%) malignancies became symptomatic [relative risk, 9.7 (95% CI, 1.3–36.8; $P < 0.01$]. Overall, malignancies identified in the extensive screening group were at an earlier stage and the mean delay to diagnosis was reduced from 11.6 to 1.0 months ($P < 0.001$). Cancer-related mortality during the 2 years follow-up period occurred in two (2.0%) of the 99 patients of the extensive screening group vs. four (3.9%) of the 102 control patients [absolute difference, 1.9% (95% CI,) 5.5–10.9)].

Rickles et al (162) stated that while migratory thrombophlebitis is a clear indicator of an underlying neoplasm, the risk of cancer in patients with the more typical form of VTE has been the subject of intense debate over recent years. The authors concluded that, the cost-effectiveness of aggressive screening for cancer in patients with VTE remains questionable.

Nordström, M et al (163) conducted a prospective study of 366 patients in Malmo, Sweden, who had treatment after positive results on venography reported an overall incidence of deep venous thrombosis of 159 per 100 000 inhabitants per year. At the time of diagnosis of deep venous thrombosis, 71 patients (19%) had a known cancer and a further 19 (5%) developed cancer within the following year. Eight of the cancers were obvious at the time of diagnosis of the deep venous thrombosis and 11 were occult.

To date, there is very little evidence that routine cancer screening is indicated or cost-effective in patients with unprovoked thrombosis. Nonetheless, it is prudent to perform a comprehensive history and physical exam and check basic blood work with relevant tumor markers, as deemed appropriate, in patients with unprovoked thrombosis because about 90% of occult cancers can be detected using this conservative approach (164-165).

At our institutions, when performing pulmonary artery CTA and CTV for unprovoked VTE, our radiologist analyzes all information produced by the imaging examination. An attentive analysis of the entire thoracic and abdominal structures on all pulmonary artery CTA and CTV examinations is routine. Careful evaluation is also made in hospitalized patients in whom thromboembolic disease is discovered incidentally. In such patients, pulmonary artery CTA and CTV is considered a cancer screening procedure with an increased likelihood of finding an occult malignancy. When the CTV examination begins at the level of the diaphragm instead of below the level of the iliac crest, it permits the detection of venous thrombosis and serves as a simultaneous screening for possible underlying malignant disease.

4. The use of biomarkers for risk assessment for VTE in cancer patients

Despite the well documented association of cancer with increased risk of thrombosis, clinical studies have not consistently demonstrated improved outcomes with thromboprophylaxis in all groups of cancer patients, and hence their risk for VTE in view of the heterogenity of cancer (166).

Moreover, treatment of VTE in patients with cancer or use of pharmacological agents for thromboprophylaxis is more difficult and is associated with considerable therapeutic challenges in view of thrombocytopenia caused by some chemotherapeutic agents and morbidity associated with VTE in often medically compromised cancer patients (32, 167)

Therefore, identification of a high-risk subgroup of cancer patients who will benefit from primary thromboprophylaxis is well justified. Recent data have identified multiple clinical risk factors as depicted under patient-, disease- and treatment-related risk factors above as well as biomarkers predictive of VTE in cancer patients. Biomarkers associated with increased risk of cancer associated VTE include leukocyte count, platelet count, and levels of tissue factor, P-selectin, D-dimer and CRP as discussed below.

a. **Leukocyte count:** Leukocytosis was identified as independent risk factor associated with increased risk of VTE in cancer patients before initiating chemotherapy (OR 2.0). VTE occurred in 4.5% patients with baseline leukocytosis, WBC $\geq 11x10^9/L$, compared to (1.8%) without leukocytosis ($p < 0.0001$). In a prospective observational study of 3303 ambulatory cancer patients: "Awareness of Neutropenia in Chemotherapy" Study Group Registry, leukocyte count $>11.0x10^9/L$ was also reported to be independently associated with an increased risk of subsequent VTE. Leukocytosis may be a marker of the aggressiveness of the cancer cells or represent a direct causative role in mediating cancer-associated thrombosis, through, as yet, unknown mechanisms (168-169).
b. **Platelet count:** Thrombocytosis is often observed in cancer patients and elevated platelet counts correlates with an activation of coagulation. In several studies of cancer patients, an elevated platelet count ($\geq 350x10^9/l$) prior to starting chemotherapy was found to be strongly associated with VTE (21, 19). The incidence of VTE was 4-7.9% in patients with a pre-chemotherapy platelet count $\geq 350x10^9/l$ compared to 1.25% in patients with lower platelet counts. The increased risk of VTE with higher platelet counts persisted while the patients were on chemotherapy and these patients had a 3-fold higher rate of VTE (32).
c. **D-Dimer** is a degradation product of cross-linked fibrin that is formed after thrombin-generated fibrin clots have been degraded by plasmin. Elevated fibrin D-dimer level (HR, 1.8) and elevated prothrombin split products (HR, 2.0) have recently been shown to be associated with increased risk of VTE in a large prospective study of cancer patients (170). D-dimer was also elevated in metastatic breast cancer patients compared to normal controls (171). These and other data suggest that D-dimer levels may be a predictor of VTE in cancer patients.
d. **Clotting factor VIII (VIII:C)** This factor plays an important role in the coagulation cascade. In non-cancer patients, a high FVIII: C activity has been established as a risk factor for primary and recurrent VTE (25-26, 51). In a prospective cohort study, a significant association was found between FVIII:C levels and the risk of symptomatic VTE in cancer patients (51). In an analysis of cancer patients including solid cancers and haematological malignancies, the cumulative probability of VTE after 6 months was 14% in patients with elevated FVIII (cut-off: 232%) as opposed to 4% in those with normal levels ($p = 0.001$). These results demonstrate that elevated FVIII:C levels in cancer patients proved to be a valuable, independent risk marker for VTE, predicting an

almost 3-fold increased VTE risk **(172).** Cumulative probability of VTE after 6 months was 14% in patients with elevated FVIII:C levels

e. **The prothrombin fragment** 1+2 (F1+2) is released when activated factor X cleaves prothrombin to thrombin and reflects the in-vivo thrombin generation. A systematic activation of coagulation has been observed in cancer patients which is reflected by elevated plasma levels of global coagulation markers, such as D-Dimer or prothrombin fragment 1+2 (F1+2) (49, 173).
f. **Tissue factor (TF)** is a transmembrane glycoprotein present on subendothelial tissue, platelets, and leukocytes that initiates coagulation and plays a critical role in regulating hemostasis and thrombosis (174-175). TF expression has been shown to be associated with increased angiogenesis in various solid neoplasms, including hepatocellular, colorectal and prostate cancers as well as in haematologic malignancies and play a role in cancer-associated thrombosis (176-177). TF induction was shown to be an early event in the development of pancreatic cancer and that the level of TF expression correlates with increased angiogenesis and with subsequent development of symptomatic VTE (176-179).

VTE was 4-fold more common ($p = 0.04$) among patients with high TF-expressing carcinomas (20%) than among those with low TF-expressing carcinomas (5.5%). There is a potential for circulating TF to be used as predictive biomarker for pancreatic cancer associated VTE. VTE was 4-fold more common ($p = 0.04$) among patients with high TF-expressing carcinomas (26.5%) than among those with low TF-expressing carcinomas (5.5%). In another study, TF expression correlated with subsequent VTE in a series of patients with ovarian cancer (173).

Furthermore, a retrospective analysis of cancer patients without VTE, revealed a 1-year cumulative incidence of VTE of 34.8% in patients with TF-bearing MPs versus 0% in those without detectable TF-bearing MPs ($p= 0.002$).

g. **Soluble P-selectin (sPS):** This is a cell adhesion molecule found in the membranes of platelets and endothelial cells (Weibel–Palade bodies) where it can function as a receptor and mediate cell adhesion via binding to several ligands. The interaction of sPS with PSGL-1 expressed on the majority of leukocytes results in the release of procoagulant, tissue factor-rich microparticles (MPs) from leukocytes, endothelial cells, platelets and cancer cells (179). In case-control studies of non-cancer patients with a history of VTE and healthy subjects without a history of venous or arterial thrombosis, high plasma levels of sPS have been demonstrated to be strongly associated with VTE (27, 35). In a multivariate analysis of the prospective observational Vienna Cancer and Thrombosis Study, elevated sPS (cutoff level, 53.1 mg/mL) was a statistically significant risk factor for VTE after adjustment for age, sex, surgery, chemotherapy and radiotherapy (HR = 2.6) and the cumulative probability of VTE after 6 months was 11.9% in patients with high sPS and 3.7% in those normal levels ($p = .002$) (180).

C- Reactive Protein

C-reactive protein (CRP) is an inflammatory marker produced by the liver and adipocytes. In a prospective study, CRP was significantly associated with increased risk of VTE by multivariate analysis (181-183)

		Factor
CLINICAL RISK FACTORS	Patient Related Factors	• Age - > 60 years • Gender • Race • Previous thrombotic episode • Obesity: BMI ≥ 35 kg/m^2 • Chronic co-morbid Medical Conditions
	Disease Related Factors	• Tumors type • Initial cancer stage • Biological aggressiveness of cancer • Rate of metastatic spread
	Treatment Related Factors	• Chemotherapy • Anti-angiogenic and immunomodulatory agents • Use of Hemopoetic growth factors • Surgery • Indwelling central venous catheters • Radiation • Hormonal therapy
BIOMARKERS	Biomarkers	• Leukocyte count ≥ $11x10^9/L$ • Platelet count ≥ 350 $x10^9/L$ • D-Dimer • Clotting factor VIII • The prothrombin fragment • Tissue factor (TF) • Soluble P-selectin • C-Reactive protein

Table 1. Summary of the Risk Factors for VTE in Cancer Patients

5. VTE in haematological malignancies

Although the association between malignancy and thrombosis has been well recognized, less is known about the risk of thrombosis in patients with acute leukemia and the impact of VTE on survival. Certainly there is abundant biochemical evidence for thrombin generation and disseminated intravascular coagulation in patients with leukemia (184). The few single-center reports of the incidence of venous thrombosis in patients with leukaemia have focused primarily on children with acute lymphoblastic leukaemia. These studies have suggested the cumulative incidence varies between 2% and 10.6% (185-186).

Patients with haematologic malignancies are at high risk of thrombotic or haemorrhagic complications. The incidence of VTE events varies considerably and is influenced by many factors, including the type of disease, chemotherapy used, and whether a central venous device is inserted. As in solid tumors, a number of clinical risk factors have been identified and contribute to the increasing thrombotic rate in haematologic malignancies. Biologic properties of the tumor cells can influence the hypercoagulable state of patients with these malignancies by several mechanisms. Of interest, oncogenes responsible for haematological neoplastic transformation in leukemia also may be involved in haemostatic activation.

- **VTE in Central Nervous System Lymphoma**

Patients with brain tumors are at particularly high risk for VTE, and many studies found that the hazard for deep vein thrombosis in patients with malignant glioma may reach 28% (187-188) This high risk is maintained throughout the course of an active disease and during treatment, and not just in the immediate postoperative period (188). Risk factors for VTE in patients with glioma include the presence of paraparesis, a histologic diagnosis of glioblastoma multiforme, age ≥ 60 years, large tumor size, the use of chemotherapy, and length of surgery of > 4 hours. Because of the high incidence of VTE, patients who are treated for brain tumors are usually considered for long term prophylactic anticoagulation as deemed appropriate for a particular patient (189-190).

- **VTE in Non-Hodgkin Lymphoma**

The incidence of clinical VTE in patients with malignant lymphoma reportedly ranges between 6.6% and 13.3% (187, 190-194) In one study, 50% of patients had a bulky tumor compressing a vein, 25% of patients had a central catheter at the thrombosed vein, and, in the other patients, thrombosis was attributed to paraneoplasia or to chemotherapy (187)

Conlon SJ et al (194) reported the results of retrospective analysis of patients with a total of 18 653 cases on the NCI Working Formulation: there were 5496 low grade NHL, 12 251 aggressive NHL and 906 high-grade lymphoma cases. The cumulative incidence (CI) of VTE 24 months from diagnosis was 4.0%. The CI of VTE at 24 months were significantly different for the distinct lymphoma groups (p< 0.001, Chi-square and comparisons showed this difference to be significant only between the low grade and other histologies. Of 742 cases that had VTE, 454 died within 2 years (61%). For those without VTE, 7274 of 17911 (41%) died within 2 years. This difference was statistically significant (p < 0.001, Chi-square).

- **VTE In Patient with Acute Leukemia**

A population- based cohort study (1993-1999) to determine the incidence and risk factors associated with development of VTE among Californians diagnosed with acute leukemia (1993-1999) was reported in Blood 2009, by Ku GH et al (195). Among 5394 cases of AML, the 2-year cumulative incidence of VTE was 281 (5.2%) and 64% of VTE events occurred within 3 months of AML diagnosis. The authors reported that, in AML patients, female sex, older age, number of co-morbid conditions, presence of CVC were significant predictors for development of VTE within one year following diagnosis of acute leukemia but the event of VTE was not associated with poor survival in AML patients in the studied group. Among 2482 case of ALL, the 2-year incidence of VTE was 4.5% and risk factors in this group were presence of CVC, older age and number of chronic co-morbidities. In this study, development of VTE in ALL patients was associated with a 40% increase of dying within one year.

In the abstract #6595 published in JCO 2011 by Luong NV et al from MD Anderson Cancer Center, USA (196) of a retrospective chart review to determine the prevalence of VTE prior to treatment and recurrence of VTE. Records of 299 ALL patients and 996 AML patients were included (Nov 1991-May 2005). The authors concluded that acute leukemia patients have a high prevalence of VTE but the occurrence of VTE prior to initiation of chemotherapy was not associated with poor prognosis similar finding to that reported by Ku GH et al.

Blast cells with their procoagulant properties, central venous catheters, chemotherapeutic agents (as discussed earlier in this chapter) concomitant infections, patient-and supportive treatment related factors are major determinants of haemostatic mechanism activation in acute leukemia. The clinical manifestations range from VTE to diffuse life-threatening hemorrhage. Anti-coagulant therapy in this clinical setting is fraud with major difficulties as the patients are at very high risk of haemorrhage because of thrombocytopenia. To date, no guidelines are available for prophylaxis or treatment of VTE in this group of patients (197)

- **VTE in Acute Promyelocytic Leukemia**

The use of the differentiating agent all-trans-retinoic acid (ATRA) in the treatment of APL allowed achievement of complete remission in more than 90% of the cases and improved dramatically the coagulopathy typical of this disease (198). The modifications induced by ATRA in the balance between procoagulant and fibrinolytic properties of the pathological promyelocytes before complete differentiation have been proposed to induce a prothrombotic effect (199).

- **VTE in Multiple Myeloma**

Multiple myeloma (MM) has been associated with increased risk of VTE events. Specific risk factors for VTE in MM are production of autoantibodies to haemostatic factors, high incidence of acquired protein C resistance, increased VIII:C levels and VWF and increase of production of inflammatory cytokines e.g. IL-6, TNF and C-reactive protein and paraprotein. These unique risk factors may operate along other common cancer VTE risk factors e.g. age, immobility, cancer procoagulant factors and chemotherapy.

Treatment regimens for MM include thalidomide, Lenalidomide combined with glucocorticoids and cytotoxic chemotherapy are associated with an increased risk of VTE particularly when the immunomodulatory agents are combined with anthracyclines. Combination chemotherapy including thalidomide plus dexamethasone and/or alkylating agents are associated with intermediate risk for VTE. The use of newer immunomodulator e.g. bortezomib seem to reduce the VTE risk **(200).** This topic has been well covered in chapter 5 of the book.

- **VTE in Monoclonal gammopathy of undetermined significance**

In 2004, Sallah S et al and Srkalovic G et al published in Ann Oncol and cancer respectively (201-202) two small hospital based studies on the association of monoclonal gammopathy of undetermined significance (MGUS) and subsequent risk of DVT and reported an elevated risk of DVT in MGUS. Kristinsson Y et al (203) conducted a retrospective study on 4,196,197 veterans hospitalized at least once. MM was identified in 2374 (0.06%) cases of MGUS 6192 (0.15%). A total of 31 and 151 DVTs occurred among MGUS and multiple myeloma, respectively (crude incidence 31 and 8.7 per 1000 person-years, respectively). The RR of DVT after a diagnosis of MGUS and MM was 3.3 and 9.2 respectively with excess risk of DVT in the first year of diagnosis. Compared to the background population, patients with multiple myeloma have a 9-fold increased risk of developing DVT especially during the first year of diagnosis while the risk for DVT in MGUS was stable at 3-fold increased risk over time with no statistical association between DVT in MGUS and risk for progression into MM.

- **VTE in Myelodysplastic Syndrome**

Yang X et al (204), in 2009, reported a total of 7764 MDS patient who were prescribed Lenalidomide during the first two years of its commercial use in the USA. VTE was reported in 41 patients (rate of 0.53%) denoting a computed signal that did not exceed the statistical threshold for identification of a significant disproportional signal for VTE in MDS on Lenalidomide without erythropoietin. However, the authors found that a disproportional signal of VTE where erythropoietin was concurrently administered with Lenalidomide.

- **VTE in Myeloproliferative Neoplasms**

Life expectancy of patients with myeloproliferative neoplasms (MPNs) and particularly that of subjects with polycythemia vera (PV) and essential thrombocythemia (ET) has significantly increased over the last three decades, largely due to the use of cytoreductive treatments. Currently, PRV and ET are considered relatively benign diseases in which the main objective of treatment strategy is the prevention of thrombotic events. Widespread use of routine haematologic screening and novel diagnostic tools greatly facilitate disease recognition and treatment. This helps to prevent a significant number of early vascular events that still constitute the first disease manifestation in approximately one-third of patients (205). We can also expect that new therapeutic options and appropriate use of aspirin will result in a further reduction of morbidity and mortality. One of the unmet needs of PRV and ET is validated methods for vascular risk stratification. The evaluation of the thrombotic risk in the individual patients, as reported by Barbui et al. in their paper (206).

The pathogenesis of thrombosis in myeloproliferative neoplasms has been extensively investigated by focusing in particular on the possible contribution of disease related haemostatic abnormalities. However, the pathogenesis of thrombosis appears to be multifactorial. Red blood cell, platelet, and leukocyte abnormalities, both qualitative and quantitative, are likely to play a key-role in myeloproliferative neoplasm thrombophilia. High shear stress of the vessel wall, due to blood hyperviscosity, accounts for chronic endothelial dysfunction and platelet and leukocyte activation.

Platelets and endothelial cells play a pivotal role in regulating blood flow, both cells might contribute to determine a prothrombotic microenvironment in myeloproliferative neoplasm patients by producing more soluble selectins and less nitric oxide, likely as a consequence of inflammation (207).

According to the data of Barbui et al. (208) it is intriguing to consider the possibility that pentraxin 3 response to inflammation in subjects with high JAK2 burden might contribute to lower or enhance the thrombotic risk. More generally the association between JAK2 mutation, inflammation and thrombotic risk deserves scientific attention also for other speculative and practical purposes.

6. The scoring system for risk assessment for VTE in cancer patients

The development of predictive risk assessment model in non-cancer patients has helped to stratify patients according to their VTE risk and tailor thromboprophylaxis accordingly. Some models in surgical patients stratified patients according to the type of operation (major or minor), age and the presence of additional risk factors eg. cancer, prior VTE, obesity, co-morbid medical conditions.

In cancer patients, risk stratification is a dynamic process depending on the type and stage of cancer, performance status, and supportive and specific cancer therapy. A model-based approach that incorporates multiple risk factors for VTE can help identify the high-risk subgroups in the cancer population and would allow for a directed prophylactic strategy to improve outcomes of management and sparing the low risk patients from unnecessary anticoagulation therapy with its complications, social and financial burden. The ideal score model has to be simple, sensitive, specific and well validated.

Khorana AA et al (209) developed a simple model for predicting chemotherapy-associated VTE using baseline clinical and laboratory variables. The association of VTE with multiple variables was characterized in a derivation cohort of 2701 cancer outpatients from a prospective observational study. A risk model was derived and validated in an independent cohort of 1365 patients from the same study. Five (2 clinical and 3 laboratory) predictive variables were identified in a multivariate model: site of cancer (2 points for very high-risk site, 1 point for high-risk site), platelet count of ≥350 × 10^9/L, Hb <100 g/L (10 g/dL) and/or use of erythropoiesis-stimulating agents, WBC ≥11 × 10^9/L, and BMI of ≥35 kg/m2 or more (1 point each). Rates of VTE in the derivation and validation cohorts, respectively, were 0.8% and 0.3% in low-risk (score = 0), 1.8% and 2% in intermediate-risk (score = 1-2), and 7.1% and 6.7% in high-risk (score ≥ 3) category over a median of 2.5 months (C-statistic = 0.7 for both cohorts). Khorana AA et al stated that their model can identify patients with a nearly 7% short-term risk of symptomatic VTE.

Patients characteristics	Risk score
Site of Cancer	
Very high risk (stomach, pancreas)	2
High risk (lung, lymphoma, gynecologic, bladder, testicular)	1
Prechemotherapy platelet count ≥ 350x10/L	1
Hemoglobin level ≤ 10g/dl or use or erythropoietin	1
Prechemotherapy leukocyte count more than 11000/mm^3	1
Body mass index 35 kg/m^2 or more	1

Table 2. Predictive model for chemotherapy-associated VTE
Adapted from Khorana et al. (209) with permission

To improve prediction of VTE in cancer patients, Ay C et al (210) performed a prospective and observational cohort study of patients with newly diagnosed cancer or progression of disease after remission. Khorana's risk scoring model for prediction of VTE that included clinical (tumor entity and body mass index) and laboratory (Hb, platelet and WBC count) parameters was expanded by incorporating 2 biomarkers, soluble P-selectin, and D-Dimer.

Of 819 patients 61 (7.4%) experienced VTE during a median follow-up of 656 days. The cumulative VTE probability in the original risk model after 6 months was 17.7% in patients with the highest risk score (≥ 3, n = 93), 9.6% in those with score 2 (n = 221), 3.8% in those with score 1 (n = 229) and 1.5% in those with score 0 (n = 276). In the expanded risk model, the cumulative VTE probability after 6 months in patients with the highest score (≥ 5, n = 30) was 35.0% and 10.3% in those with an intermediate score (score 3, n = 130) as opposed to only 1.0% in patients with score 0 (n = 200); the hazard ratio of patients with the highest compared with those with the lowest score was 25.9 (8.0-84.6). The authors demonstrated that clinical and standard laboratory parameters with addition of biomarkers enable prediction of VTE and allow identification of cancer patients at high or low risk of VTE.

Ay C et al concluded that with expanded risk model, which included sP-selectin ≥53.1 mg/ml and D-Dimer ≥1.44 mg/ml, (2 biomarkers) the risk prediction can be considerably improved. In patients with the highest compared with patients with the lowest risk, the probability for VTE was 26-fold higher.

The advantage of the "Khorana-Score" is that all parameters of this risk model are routinely determined in cancer patients at diagnosis.

7. Prevention of venous thromboembolism in cancer patients

Using Khorana risk scoring model or Ay Cihan et al expanded scoring model, it is within the reach of the attending hematologist/oncologist to stratify his/her cancer patient into one of the VTE risk groups: very high, high, intermediate or low and consider the patient for thromboprophylaxis in a patient-focused approach.

It also well understood that prophylaxis with antithrombotic agents can be problematic in cancer patients because they are at increased risk for anticoagulant induced bleeding. However, prophylaxis has been shown to be beneficial in certain high-risk populations such as post-surgical or hospitalized cancer patients but data in the ambulatory settings are conflicting.

7.1 Prophylaxis in surgical cancer patients

In general, surgery for cancer increases the risk of VTE and adequate prophylaxis has been shown to reduce VTE rates significantly [99,100]. A number of studies have shown that patients with cancer who undergo a specific type of major surgery have a 2-4 fold higher incidence of postoperative VTE compared with patients without cancer. The risk of venographically proven DVT varies from 20% to 40% and the risk of fatal PE is approximately 1%. Therefore, routine prophylaxis with anticoagulant therapy is strongly recommended, both in the immediate post-operative setting and in the extended period following major surgery.

The agents used most widely for prophylaxis in surgical patients are unfractionated heparin (UFH) and low-molecular- weight heparin (LMWH). Meta-analysis of randomized trials evaluating anticoagulant prophylaxis in general surgery, Mismetti et al. (211), found no significant difference between LMWH and UFH in symptomatic VTE, major bleeding, transfusion and death. This finding is supported by the ENOXACAN study (212). The

ENOXACAN II study was conducted to examine the effect extended prophylaxis i.e. 21 days, significantly reduced the incidence of DVT from 12% to 4.8% (p= 0.02).

7.2 Thromboprophylaxis in hospitalized or bedridden cancer patients

As the incidence of VTE in cancer patients who require hospitalization is very high, therefore they would benefit from primary anticoagulant prophylaxis. However, it is likely that the absolute and relative benefit of primary thromboprophylaxis will vary greatly amongst different patient groups because of the heterogeneity of cancer patient. It appears that the greatest potential impact of primary prophylaxis would be in patients initially diagnosed with advanced disease particularly those who are candidates for chemotherapy. Another subgroup of patients who may warrant primary thromboprophylaxis are patients initially diagnosed with local, or regional-stage cancer who progress and develop metastatic cancer or when they are admitted to hospital with an acute illness. Those patients should always be considered for primary pharmacological as well as mechanical thromboprophylaxis. Although none of the clinical studies evaluated a cancer-specific population, consensus statements and guidelines unanimously support the use of prophylaxis in cancer patients admitted to hospitals.

7.3 Thromboprophylaxis in ambulatory cancer patients

Much less is known about prevention of VTE in ambulatory cancer patients. The incidence of symptomatic VTE observed in ambulatory patients with advanced or metastatic malignancies in a recent clinical trial of 3% is considered low (26). Multiple recent studies have evaluated the potential benefit of thromboprophylaxis in ambulatory patients selected on the basis of one or two risk factors but have been unable to definitively identify patients who would benefit from prophylaxis

In the double-blind study by Levine et al (213) evaluated the anticoagulant effect of very low-dose warfarin (INR1.3-1.9) in Stage IV breast cancer while they were receiving chemotherapy. However, more recent trials have failed to confirm the benefit of primary prophylaxis in the ambulatory setting.

In summary, routine anticoagulant prophylaxis in medical oncology patients is not practiced because (a) the incidence of symptomatic VTE observed in ambulatory patients with advanced or metastatic malignancies is considered low. (b), the risk of bleeding remains a significant concern in most patients with cancer. (c) extended periods of primary prevention with an anticoagulant can be unattractive to most patients with cancer and (d) the optimal period of prophylaxis has not been identified.

One established high-risk group in the ambulatory setting is multiple myeloma patients receiving combination therapy. All newly diagnosed patients treated with thalidomide/lenalidomide- containing regimens should receive thromboprophylaxis as detailed in chapter 5.

7.4 Primary VTE prophylaxis in palliative care settings

Sarah Mclean and James S O'Donnell (214) published a qualitative systemic review that covered the period (1960-2010) on this important aspect of management of cancer patients

(Palliative Medicine June 2010). The authors pointed that primary thromboprophylaxis with LMWH is under utilized in the palliative setting although it is supported by level 1A evidence. The authors stated that studies examined practice in specialist patient care units and attitude held by a total of 32 palliative care physicians and 198 patients for thromboprophylaxis revealed that patient perception of LMWH is based on physician's concern regarding the negative impact on quality life and lack of evidence to support such practice. The authors concluded that LMWH prophylaxis in palliative patients with previous good performance status needs further studies.

7.5 Guidelines for VTE prophylaxis in cancer patients

The recommendation of the American College of Chest Physicians (ACCP) guidelines on prevention of VTE recommends prophylaxis for acutely ill hospitalized medical/surgical patients with cancer (215). However, the compliance of oncologists with the recommendations remains low (216) and this may be due to lack of awareness or unfounded fear of bleeding within the oncology community. Institution-based VTE prophylaxis guidelines with risk for VTE stratification followed by effective monitoring and auditing policy by the institution and sustained awareness campaigns could have a significant positive impact.

The Guidelines

The reader is referred to the following rich evidence-based guidelines:

1. ACCP guidelines is an evidence-based on antithrombotic and thrombolytic therapy covering both prevention and treatment with selected issues related to cancer patients (http://www.chestnet.org/accp/)
2. National Comprehensive Cancer Network (NCCN), a non-profit, alliance of 20 leading National Cancer Institute-designated Cancer Centers. The NCCN develops and disseminates clinical practice guidelines in oncology. The latest version of recommendations on VTE management can be found on-line at nccn.org/professionals/physicians_gls/PDF/vte.pdf.
3. Italian Guidelines on Management of VTE in patients with cancer published on-line by the Italian Association of Medical Oncologists for Italian oncologists. The guideline covers different aspects of VTE and cancer (a) VTE associated with occult malignancies (b) prophylaxis in cancer surgery, during chemotherapy, during hormonal therapy (c) VTE prophylaxis of VTE associated central venous catheters (d) treatment of VTE in cancer patients (e) anticoagulation and prognosis of cancer. The Italian recommendations are updated annually.
4. The American Society of Clinical Oncology Guidelines published its latest recommendations for VTE prophylaxis and treatment in patients with cancer in Dec 2007, JCD volume 25, No. 34 (5490-5505). Our reader is encouraged to refer to this informative and comprehensive document. The ASCO recommendations are depicted in a user-friendly practical approach in a format of practical questions.
   1. Should hospitalized patients with cancer receive anticoagulation for VTE prophylaxis?
   2. Should ambulatory patients with cancer receive anticoagulation for VTE during systematic chemotherapy?

3. Should patients with cancer undergoing surgery receive preoperative VTE prophylaxis?
4. What is the best treatment for patients with cancer with established VTE to prevent recurrent VTE?
5. Should patients with cancer receive anticoagulants in the absence of established VTE to improve survival?

8. Consequences of cancer-associated thrombosis

As depicted above in this chapter, the implications of diagnosis of VTE in a patient with cancer are many:

a. Mortality: cancer diagnosed at the same as or within a year of an episode of VTE is associated with 3-fold increase in mortality at one year. Moreover, the mortality rate in hospitalized cancer patients is higher when they develop VTE. For ambulatory cancer patients, initiating treatment with chemotherapy, VTE and arterial thrombosis has been reported to account for 9% of death. The risk of dying from fatal PE in cancer patient undergoing surgery is 3-fold higher than similar surgery in non-cancer patients.
b. Bleeding complications: cancer patients with VTE and treated with anticoagulants are at two-fold greater risk of bleeding complications than patients with VTE but no cancer.
c. Negative impact on healthcare resources: in a retrospective study Etting LS et al (Arch Int Med 2008) reported that the average cost of hospitalization for the index DVT episode in cancer patients in USA was $20065 in 2002 and the attributable hospital stay was 11 days.
d. Recurrence rate of VTE in a patient with cancer is 3-fold more frequently than in patients without cancer. Prandoni et al (32) performed a prospective cohort study of consecutive patients with incident VTE and compared the incidence of recurrence and bleeding for those with and without cancer at the time of VTE. Patients were given heparin followed by warfarin. The 12-month cumulative incidence of recurrent VTE in the group with cancer was 20.7% (95% CI 15.6-25.8%) vs. 6.8% (95% CI 3.9-9.7%) in those without malignancy. The rate of recurrence was directly associated with tumor burden as prospectively assessed by the investigators. This study also confirmed that the risk of major bleeding was also higher for patients with extensive cancer on warfarin anticoagulation. Compared to patients without cancer, patients with cancer have a higher risk of thrombosis and recurrent thrombosis. Recent evidence from well-conducted clinical trials shows that cancer patients may benefit from a longer duration of prophylaxis after surgery and that treatment with long-term LMWH is more effective than conventional oral anticoagulant therapy. Randomized studies have shown that prolonged (6 months) treatment with LMWH results in both lower VTE recurrence rates and less bleeding. Thus, LMWH is the therapy of choice for treatment of VTE in patients with cancer. However, the optimal duration of therapy for patients with active cancer has not been determined.
e. Post-Thrombotic Syndrome

Available data on the incidence of post-thrombotic syndrome in patients with cancer is scarce. However, approximately 30% of patients with DVT subsequently develop this chronic, frequently disabling condition within 5 years of the event. Of those, 8.1% will have severe post-thrombotic manifestations (Prandoni et al, 1997b) (8). It is expected that the incidence of the syndrome in cancer patients would be higher in view of adverse patient and treatment related factors. Symptoms of post-thrombotic syndrome include debilitating leg pain, swelling, and fibrosis. Severe manifestations may result in debilitating leg ulceration, mobility problems, and the need for long-term nursing care.

f. Pulmonary Hypertension

Pulmonary hypertension is a life-threatening condition associated with fatigue, chest pain, peripheral swelling, and increased mortality. Recent studies suggest that 4–5% of patients develop pulmonary hypertension within years after symptomatic PE, Pengo et al, 2004 (216).

9. Treatment of VTE

Several studies have addressed treatment of VTE in patients with cancer:

a. The CLOT (Comparison of Low-Molecular-Weight Heparin Versus Oral Anticoagulant Therapy for the Prevention of Recurrent Venous Thromboembolism in Patients with Cancer, N Engl J Med. 2003) study, which compared dalteparin with vitamin K antagonist (VKA) therapy, is the largest randomized trial of VTE treatment in patients with cancer (n = 672) (183). This study reported a 52% RRR in the incidence of recurrent VTE in favor of dalteparin during the 6-month study period.
b. Three additional studies assessed the use of LMWH for extended VTE treatment in patients with cancer. The CANTHANOX (Secondary Prevention Trial of Venous Thrombosis with Enoxaparin) study compared 3 months of warfarin therapy with 3 months of enoxaparin therapy in patients with malignancy and proximal DVT or PE (218). Because of slow recruitment, the study was terminated prematurely. At 3 months, seven patients in the enoxaparin group had recurrent VTE or major bleeding (the combined primary end point) versus 15 patients in the warfarin group (P = 0.09). Most of the primary outcomes were due to major bleeding (five patients in the enoxaparin group versus 12 in the warfarin group). In the warfarin group, six of the patients died of major bleeding, and at the 6-month follow-up, 31% of patients in the enoxaparin group had died, compared with 38.7% of patients in the warfarin group (P = 0.25). The findings of this limited study suggest that warfarin may be associated with a higher risk of bleeding than LMWH when used as long-term VTE treatment in patients with cancer (218).
c. The three-arm ONCENOX (Secondary Prevention Trial of Venous Thrombosis with Enoxaparin) study included 101 patients with cancer and VTE. Because of the small number of patients enrolled, no differences between the enoxaparin and warfarin groups were observed with regard to the incidence of recurrent VTE, major bleeding, or death (219).
d. The LITE (Long-Term Innohep Treatment Evaluation) study found tinzaparin to be more efficacious than warfarin in 200 patients with cancer (220). Tinzaparin treatment reduced the rate of recurrent VTE by ~50%; however, the difference was not statistically significant at the end of the 3-month treatment period. There were no differences in bleeding rates between the two groups.

Compared with warfarin, LMWHs generally reduce the overall risk of recurrent VTE when used for the extended treatment of VTE, a finding confirmed by a recently published Cochrane systematic review (221). Furthermore, LMWHs do not increase major bleeding rates and appear to be as safe as VKAs. These findings, like those seen in the prevention trials, appear to be related to the dose and the duration of therapy.

The standard treatment for acute VTE is anticoagulant therapy. For initial therapy, subcutaneous (SC) LMWH is as effective and safe as intravenous UFH (28, 29). LMWHs are administered once or twice daily by SC injection, have weight-adjusted dosing and do not usually require laboratory monitoring. These advantages over UFH allow LMWHs to be given on an outpatient basis and reduce the need for hospitalization.

Duration of therapy: Duration of anticoagulant therapy has not been addressed in cancer patients. Based on the accepted concept that the risk of recurrent thrombosis is increased in the presence of any ongoing risk factor, it is generally recommended that patients with metastases continue with "indefinite" therapy because metastatic malignancy is a persistent risk factor. In those without metastases, anticoagulant treatment is recommended for as long as the cancer is "active" and while the patient is receiving antitumor therapy.

Secondary prophylaxis: Oral anticoagulant therapy with a vitamin K antagonist can be started on the same day as heparin therapy to begin secondary prophylaxis. To effectively reduce recurrent VTE without excessive bleeding, the dose of oral anticoagulants must be adjusted to maintain the INR within a therapeutic range of 2.0 to 3.0. This usually requires twice weekly blood work for the first 1 to 2 weeks until a stable dose is identified. Using this regimen, the annual incidence of recurrent VTE in patients without cancer is approximately 8%, whereas the risk of recurrence is two- to threefold higher in patients with cancer.

The higher failure rate in cancer patients may reflect the greater difficulty in maintaining therapeutic INR levels because of multiple drug interactions, gastrointestinal upset, vitamin K deficiency, liver dysfunction and poor venous access. Also, temporary discontinuation of anticoagulant therapy is often necessary during periods of thrombocytopenia and to accommodate invasive procedures. Such interruptions can cause lengthy periods of inadequate anticoagulation because vitamin K antagonists have a delayed onset of action and a prolonged period of clearance. Furthermore, warfarin failure, i.e. recurrent VTE despite maintaining therapeutic INR levels, is not uncommonly reported in cancer patients on oral anticoagulant therapy.

10. References

[1] Miller GJ, Bauer KA, Howarth DJ, Cooper JA, Humphries SE, Rosenberg RD. Increased incidence of neoplasia of the digestive tract in men with persistent activation of the coagulant pathway. J Thromb Haemost (2004) 2: 2107–2114.

[2] Hoffman R, Haim N, Brenner B. Cancer and thrombosis revisited. Blood Rev (2001) 15: 61–67.

[3] Oleksowicz L, Bhagwati N, DeLeon-Fernandez M. Deficient activity of von Willebrand's factor-cleaving protease in patients with disseminated malignancies. Cancer Res (1999) 59: 2244–2250.

[4] Kakkar AK, DeRuvo N, Chinswangwatanakul V, Tebbutt S, Williamson RC. Extrinsic-pathway activation in cancer with high factor VIIa and tissue factor. Lancet (1995) 346: 1004–1005.

[5] Rickles FR, Brenner B. B Tissue factor and cancer. Semin Thromb Hemost (2008) 34: 143-145.

[6] Falanga A, Gordon SG. Isolation and characterization of cancer procoagulant: a cysteine proteinase from malignant tissue. Biochemistry (1985) 24: 5558–5567.

[7] Mielicki WP, Tenderenda M, Rutkowski P, Chojnowski K. Activation of blood coagulation and the activity of cancer procoagulant (EC 3.4.22.26) in breast cancer patients. Cancer Lett (1999) 146: 61–66.

[8] Prandoni P, Villalta S, Bagatella P, Rossi L, Marchiori A, Piccoli A, Bernardi E, Girolami B, Simioni P, Girolam A. The clinical course of deep-vein thrombosis. Prospective long-term follow-up of 528 symptomatic patients. Haematologica (1997b) 82: 423-428.

[9] Qi J, Kreutzer DL. Fibrin activation of vascular endothelial cells. Induction of IL-8 expression. J Immunol (1995) 155: 867–876.

[10] Fernandez PM, Patierno SR, Rickles FR. Tissue factor and fibrin in tumor angiogenesis. Semin Thromb Hemost (2004) 30: 31–44.

[11] Rao LV, Pendurthi UR . Tissue factor-factor VIIa signaling. Arterioscler Thromb Vasc Biol (2005) 25: 47–56.

[12] Bouillard JB, Bouillaud S. Del'Obliferation de reines et de son influence sur la formation des hydro partielles: consideration sur la hydropisies passive et general Arch Gen Med 1823 1: 188-204

[13] Trousseau A, Bazire PV, Cormack JR. Lectures on Clinical Medicine. London: R. Hardwicke, 1867.

[14] Khorana AA. Malignancy, thrombosis and Trousseau: The case for an eponym. J Thromb Haemost 2003;1(12):2463 65.

[15] Silverstein MD, Heit JA, Mohr DN, Petterson TM, O'Fallon WM, Melton III LJ. Trends in the incidence of deep vein thrombosis and pulmonary embolism: a 25-year population-based study. Arch Intern Med 1998;158(6):585- 93.

[16] Gomes MP, Deitcher SR. Diagnosis of venous thromboembolic disease in cancer patients. Oncology (Huntington) 2003;17(1): 126 35, 139; discussion: 139 44.

[17] Lee AY, Levine MN. Venous thromboembolism and cancer: Risks and outcomes. Circulation 2003;107(23 Suppl 1):I17 21.

[18] Blom JW, Doggen CJ, Osanto S, Rosendaal FR. Malignancies, prothrombotic mutations, and the risk of venous thrombosis. JAMA 2005;293(6):715–22.

[19] Baron JA, Gridley G, Weiderpass E, et al. Venous thromboembolism and cancer. Lancet 1998;351(9109):1077 80.

[20] Sallah S, Wan JY, Nguyen NP. Venous thrombosis in patients with solid tumors: determination of frequency and characteristics. Thromb Haemost 2002;87(4): 575–9.

[21] Stein PD, Beemath A, Meyers FA, Skaf E, Sanchez J, Olson RE. Incidence of venous thromboembolism in patients hospitalized with cancer. Am J Med 2006;119(1): 60-8.

[22] Khorana AA, Francis CW, Culakova E, Kuderer NM, Lyman GH. Thromboembolism is a leading cause of death in cancer patients receiving outpatient chemotherapy. J Thromb Haemost 2007;5(3):632–4.

[23] Ottinger H, Belka C, Kozole G, et al. Deep venous thrombosis and pulmonary artery embolism in high-grade non Hodgkin's lymphoma: Incidence, causes and prognostic relevance. Eur J Haematol 1995;54(3):186 94.

[24] Alcalay A, Wun T, Khatri V, et al. Venous thromboembolism in patients with colorectal cancer: incidence and effect on survival. J Clin Oncol 2006;24:1112–1118. [PubMed: 16505431]

[25] Rodriguez AO, Wun T, Chew H, Zhou H, Harvey D, White RH. Venous thromboembolism in ovarian cancer. Gynecol Oncol 2007;105:784–790. [PubMed: 17408726]

[26] Chew HK, Davies AM, Wun T, Harvey D, Zhou H, White RH. The incidence of venous thromboembolism among patients with primary lung cancer. J Thromb Haemost 2008;6:601–608.PubMed: 18208538]

[27] Chew HK, Wun T, Harvey D, Zhou H, White RH. Incidence of venous thromboembolism and its effect on survival among patients with common cancers. Arch Intern Med 2006;166:458–464. [PubMed:16505267]

[28] Cavo M, Zamagni E, Cellini C, et al. Deep-vein thrombosis in patients with multiple myeloma receiving first-line thalidomide dexamethasone therapy. Blood 2002;100(6): 2272 3.

[29] Falanga A, Marchetti M. Venous thromboembolism in the hematologic malignancies. J Clin Oncol 2009 Oct 10;27(29):4848–57.

[30] Eby C. Pathogenesis and management of bleeding and thrombosis in plasma cell dyscrasias. Br J Haematol 2009 Apr;145(2):151–63.

[31] Elliott MA, Wolf RC, Hook CC, et al. Thromboembolism in adults with acute lymphoblastic leukemia during induction with L-asparaginase-containing multi-agent regimens: incidence, risk factors, and possible role of antithrombin. Leuk Lymphoma 2004;45:1545–1549. [PubMed: 15370205].

[32] Prandoni P, Lensing AW, Piccioli A, et al. Recurrent venous thromboembolism and bleeding complications during anticoagulant treatment in patients with cancer and venous thrombosis. Blood 2002;100(10):3484 8.

[33] Chew HK, Wun T, Harvey DJ, Zhou H, White RH. Incidence of venous thromboembolism and the impact on survival in breast cancer patients. J Clin Oncol 2007;25:70–76. [PubMed: 17194906]

[34] Sorensen HT, Mellemkjaer L, Olsen JH, et al. Prognosis of cancers associated with venous thromboembolism. N Engl J Med 2000;343(25):1846 50.

[35] Khorana AA, Francis CW, Culakova E, Fisher RI, Kuderer NM, Lyman GH. Thromboembolism in hospitalized neutropenic cancer patients. J Clin Oncol 2006;24(3):484–90.

[36] Khorana A. Approaches to risk-stratifying cancer patients for venous thromboembolism Thrombosis Research (2007) 120 Suppl. 2, S41–S50

[37] Agnelli G, Bolis G, Capussotti L, Scarpa RM, Tonelli F, Bonizzoni E, et al. A clinical outcome-based prospective study on venous thromboembolism after cancer surgery: the @RISTOS project. Ann Surg 2006;243:89–95.

[38] Khorana AA, Francis CW, Culakova E, Kuderer NM, Lyman GH. Frequency, risk factors, and trends for venous thromboembolism among hospitalized cancer patients. Cancer 2007;110(10):2339–46.

[39] Samama MM. An epidemiologic study of risk factors for deep vein thrombosis in medical outpatients: the Sirius study. Arch Int Med 2000;160:3415–20.

[40] Kendal WS. Dying with cancer: the influence of age, comorbidity, and cancer site. Cancer 2008;112:1354–1362. [PubMed: 18286532]

[41] Khorana AA, Francis CW, Culakova E, Kuderer NM, Lyman GH. Thromboembolism is a leading cause of death in cancer patients receiving outpatient chemotherapy. J Thromb Haemost 2007;5(3):632–4.

[42] Blom JW, Vanderschoot JP, Oostindier MJ, Osanto S, van der Meer FJ, Rosendaal FR. Incidence of venous thrombosis in a large cohort of 66,329 cancer patients: results of a record linkage study. J Thromb Haemost 2006;4:529–535. [PubMed: 16460435]

[43] White, RH;Wun, T. The burden of cancer-associated venous thromboembolism and its impact on cancer survival. In: Khorana, AA.; Francis, CW., editors. Cancer-associated Thrombosis: New Findings in Translational Science, Prevention, and Treatment. New York: Informa Healthcare, USA, Inc; 2008.

[44] Tateo S, Mereu L, Salamano S, Klersy C, Barone M, Spyropoulos AC, Piovella F. Ovarian cancer and venous thromboembolic risk. Gyn Oncol. 2005;99:119–25.

[45] Otten HM, Mathijssen J, ten Cate H, et al. Symptomatic venous thromboembolism in cancer patients treated with chemotherapy: an underestimated phenomenon. Arch Intern Med 2004;164:190–194.[PubMed: 14744843]

[46] Lee AY, Levine MN. The thrombophilic state induced by therapeutic agents in the cancer patient. Semin Thromb Hemost 1999;25:137–145. [PubMed: 10357081]

[47] Haddad TC, Greeno EW. Chemotherapy-induced thrombosis. Thromb Res 2006;118:555–568.[PubMed: 16388837]

[48] Cool R, Herringon J, Wong L. "Recurrent peripheral arterial thrombosis induced by cisplatin and etoposide." *Pharmacotherapy* 2002;22 (9): 1200-4.

[49] Licciarello J, Moake J, Rudi C, Karp D, Hong W. "Elevated plasma von Willebrand factor levels and areterial occlussive complications associated with cisplatin-based chemrotherapy." *Oncology* 1985;42:296-300.

[50] Rogers II J, Murgo A, Fontana J, Raich P. "Chemotherapy for breast cancer decreases plasma protein C and S. *J. Clin Oncol* 1988;6:276-81.

[51] Ramsay N, Coccia P, Krivit W, Nesbit M, Edson J. "The effect of L-asparaginase on plasma coagulation factors in acute lymphoblastic leukemia." *Cancer* 1977;40:1398-401.

[52] Gem K, McAtee N, Murphy R, Hamilton J, Balis F, Steinberg S, et al. "Phase I and phamacokenetic study of recombinant human granulocyte-macrophage colony stimulating factor given in combination with fluorouracil plus calcium leucovorin in metastatic gastrointestinal adenocarcinoma."*J Clin Oncol* 1994; 12:560-8.

[53] Mannuci P, Bettega D, Chantarangkul V. "Effect of women." *Arch Intern Med* 1996;156:1806-10.

[54] Greeno E, Bach R, Moldow C. "Apoptosis is associated with increased cell surface tissue factor procoagulant activity."*Lab Invest* 1996; 75:281-9.

[55] Wang J, Weiss I, Svoboda K, Kwaan H. "Thrombogenic role of cells undergoing apoptosis." *Br J Haematol.*" 2001; 115:382-91.

[56] Bertoneu M, Gallo S, Lauri D, Levine M, Orr F, Buchanan M. "Chemotherapy enhances endothelial cell rectivity to platelets."*Clin Exp Metastasis* 1990;8:511-8.

[57] Mills P, Parker B, Jones V, Adler K, Perez C, Johnson S, et al."The effects of standard anthracycline-based chemotherapy on soluble iCAM-1 and vascular endothelial growth factor levels in breast cancer." *Clin Cancer Res* 2004;10-4998-5003.

[58] Togna G, Togna A, Franconi M, Caprino L. "Cisplatin triggers platelet activation."*Thromb Res* 2000;99:503-9.

[59] Folkman J. "What is the evidence that tumors are angiogenesis dependent?" *J Natl Cancer Inst* 1990;82:4-6.

[60] Weijl N, Ruttern M, Zwinderman A, Keizer J, Nooy M, Rosendaal F, et al."Thromboemlobic events during chemotherapy for germ cell cancer: a cohort study and review of the literature."*J Clin Oncol* 2000; 18(10):2169-78.

[61] Numico G, Garrone O, Dongiovanni V, Silvestri N, Colantonio I, Di Costanzo G, et al."Prospective evaluation of major vascular events in patient with nonsmall cell lung carcinoma treated with cisplatin and gemcitabine."*Cancer* 2005;103(5):994-9.

[62] Moore RA, Nelly Adel, Elyn Riedel, Manisha Bhutani, Darren R. Feldman, Nour Elise Tabbara et al. "High Incidence of Thromboembolic Events in Patients Treated With Cisplatin-Based Chemotherapy: A Large Retrospective Analysis." *JCO* 2011;29(28):3466-3473.

[63] Sallan SE, Gelber RD, Kimball V, Donnelly M, Cohen HJ. More is better! Update of Dana-Farber Cancer Institute/Children's Hospital childhood acute lymphoblastic leukemia trials. Haematol Blood Transfus 1990;33:459-466.

[64] Amylon MD, Shuster J, Pullen J. Intensive high-dose asparaginase consolidation improves survival for pediatric patients with T cell acute lymphoblastic leukemia: a Pediatric Oncology Group Study. Blood 2000;96:335-342.

[65] Raelz EA, Sulzer WL. Tolerability and efficacy of L-asparaginase therapy in pediatric patients with acute lymphoblastic leukemia. J Pediatr Hemet Oncol 2010;32:554-563.

[66] Hongo T, Okada S, Ohzeki T, et al. Low plasma levels of hemostatic proteins during the induction phase in children with acute lymphoblastic Leukemia: a retrospective study by the JACLS. Japan Association of Childhood Leukemia Study. Pediatr Int 2002;44: 293-299.

[67]CarusoV,Iacoviello,DiCastelnuovoA,Stortis,MarianiG,deGaetanoG,DonaitiMB.Thrombo tic complications in childhood acute lymphoblastic leukemia:ameta-analysis of 17 prospective studies comprising 1752 pediatric patients. Blood 2006;108:2216-2222.

[68] Grace RF, Dahlberg SE, Neuberg D, et al. The frequency and management of asparaginase-related thrombosis in paediatric and adult patients with acute lymphoblastic leukaemia treated on Dana-Farber Cancer Institute consortium protocols. Br J Haematol 2011;152:452-459.

[69] Hunault-Berger M, Chevallier P, Detain M, et al. Changes in antithrombin and fibrinogen levels during induction chemotherapy with L-asparaginase in adult patients with acute lymphoblastic leukemia or lymphoblastic lymphoma. Use of supportive coagulation therapy and clinical outcome: the CAPELAL study. Haematologica 200893:1488-1494.

[70] Goekbuget N, Baumann A, Beck J, et al. PEG-asparaginase in adult acute lymphoblastic leukemia: efficacy and feasibility analysis with increasing dose levels. Blood 2008;112(Suppl.1): Abstract 302.

[71] Rytting M, Earl M, Douer D, Muriera B, Advani A, Bleyer A. Toxicities in adults with acute lymphoblastic leukemia treated with regimens using pegasparaginase. Blood 2008; 12(Suppl. 1): Abstract 1924.

[72] Dauer D, Watkins K, Mark L, et al. Multiple doses of intravenous pegylated asparaginase with a 'pediatric-like' protocol in adults with newly diagnosed acute

lymphohlastic leukemia (ALL): toxicity, clinical outcome and low rate of anti asparaginase antibody formation. Blood 2009;114(Suppl. 1); Abstract 3082

[73] Dauer D, Yampolsky H, Cohen LJ, et al. Pharmacodynamics and safety of intravenous pegasparaginase during remission induction in adults aged 55 years or younger with newly diagnosed acute lymphoblastic leukemia. Blood 2007;109:2744-2750.

[74] Avramis V, Sencer S, Periclou AP, et al. A randomized comparison f native Escherichia coli asparaginase and polyethylene glycol conjugated asparaginase for treatment of children with newly diagnosed standard-risk acute lymphoblastic leukemia: a Children's Cancer Group study. Blood 2002;99:/ 9136-1994.

[75] Qureshi A, Mitchell C, Richards S, Ajay Vora A, Goulden N. Asparaginase-related venous thrombosis in UKALL 2003 - re-exposure to asparaginase is feasible and safe. Br J Haematol 2010;149: 410-413.

[76] Albert S, Bretscher M, Wiltsie J, O'Neill B, Witzig T. Thrombosis related to use of L-Aspariginase in adults with acute lymphoblastic leukemia: a need to consider coagulation monitoring and clotting factor replacement: Leuk lymphoma 1999; 32:489-92

[77] Gugliotta L, Mazzucconi MG, Leone G, et at. Incidence of thrombotic complications in adult patients with acute lymphoblastic Leukaemia receiving L-asparaginase during induction therapy: a retrospective study. The GIMEMA Group. Eur J Haentatol 1992;49:63- 66.

[78] Mitchell LG, Andrew M, Hanna K, et al. A prospective cohort study determining the prevalence of thrombotic events in children with acute lymphoblastic leukemia and a central venous line who are treated with L-asparaginase: results of the Prophylactic Antithrombin Replacement in Kids with Acute Lymphoblastic Leukemia Treated with Asparaginase (PARKAA) Study. Cancer 2003;97:508-516.

[79] Nowak-Gottl U, Kenet G, Mitchell LG. Thrombosis in childhood acute lymphoblastic leukaemia: epidemiology, aetiology, diagnosis, prevention and treatment, Best Pract Res Clin Haematol 2009;22:103-114.

[80] Abbott LS, Deevska M, Fernandez CV, et al. The impact of prophylactic fresh-frozen plasma and cryoprecipitate on the Incidence of central nervous system thrombosis and hemorrhage in children with acute lymphoblastic leukemia receiving asparaginase. Blood 2009;114:5146-5151.

[81] Windy Stock, Dan Douer, Daniel J, et al. Prevention and management of asparaginase/pegasparaginase associated toxicities in adults and older adolescents: recommendation of an expert panel.

[82] Cwikiel M, Zhang B, Eskilsson J, Wieslander J, Albertsson M. The influence of 5-fluorouracil on the endothelium in small arteries. Scanning Microsc, 1995;9:561–76.

[83] Hecht JR, Trarbach T, Jaeger E., Hainsworth J, Wolff R, Lloyd K, et al. A randomized double-blind placebo-controlled phase III study in patients with metastatic adenocarcinoma of the colon or rectum receiving first-line chemotherapy with oxaliplatin/5-fluorouracil/leucovorin

[84] Hurwitz H, Fehrenbacher L, Novotny W, Cartwright T, Hainsworth J, Heim W, et al. Bevacizumab plus irinotecan, fluorouracil, and leucovorin for metastatic colorectal cancer. N Engl J Med. 2004;350:2335–42.

[85] Folkman J. Angiogenesis in cancer, vascular, rheumatoid and other disease. Nat Med. 1995;1(1):27-31.

[86] Hicklin DJ, Ellis LM. Role of the vascular endothelial growth factor pathway in tumor growth and angiogenesis. J Clin Oncol.2005;23(5):1011-1027.
[87] Motzer RJ, Bukowski RM. Targeted therapy for metastatic renal cell carcinoma. J Clin Oncol.2006;24(35);5601-5608.
[88] Nalluri SR, Chu D, Keresztes R, Zhu X, Wu S. Risk of Venous Thromboembolism with the Angiogenesis Inhibitor Bevacizumab in Cance Patients. A Meta-analysis. JAMA. 2008;300(19):2277–2285, pmid:19017914.
[89] Kilickap S, Abali H, Celik I. Bevacizumab bleeding, thrombosis, and warfarin. J Clin Oncol.2003;21(18):3542.
[90] Zachary I. Signaling mechanisms mediating vascular protective actions of vascular endothelial growth factor. Am J Physiol Cell Physiol.2001;280(6):C1375-1386.
[91] Hesser BA, Liang XH, Camenisch G, et al. Down syndrome critical region protein 1 (DSCR 1), a novel VEGF target gene that regulates expression of inflammatory markers on activated endothelial cells. Blood. 2004;104(1)149-158.
[92] Tam BY, Wei K, Rudge JS, et al. VEGF modulates erythropoiesis through regulation of adult hepatic erythropoietin synthesis. Nat Med.2006;12(7):793-800.
[93] Fein DA, Lee WR, Hanlon AL, et al. Pretreatment hemoglobin level influences local control and survival of T1–T2 squamous cell carcinomas of the glottic larynx. J Clin Oncol. 1995; 13: 2077–2083.PubMed,CAS,Web of Science® Times Cited: 1426
[94] Bush RS, Jenkin RD, Allt WE, et al. Definitive evidence for hypoxic cells influencing cure in cancer therapy. Br J Cancer. 1978; 37 (Suppl): 302–306.Web of Science® Times Cited: 4217
[95] Grogan M, Thomas GM, Melamed I, et al. The importance of hemoglobin levels during radiotherapy for carcinoma of the cervix. Cancer. 1999; 86: 1528–1536.Direct Link:AbstractFull Article (HTML)PDF(121K)References8
[96] Adamson J. Erythropoietin, iron metabolism, and red blood cell production. Semin Hematol. 1996; 33: 5–7.PubMed,CAS,Web of Science® Times Cited: 99
[97] Glaspy J, Bukowski R, Steinberg D, Taylor C, Tchekmedyian S, Vadhan-Raj S. Impact of therapy with epoetin alfa on clinical outcomes in patients with nonmyeloid malignancies during cancer chemotherapy in community oncology practice. Procrit Study Group. J Clin Oncol. 1997; 15: 1218–1234.PubMed,CAS,Web of Science® Times Cited: 46510
[98] Groopman JE, Itri LM. Chemotherapy-induced anemia in adults: incidence and treatment. J Natl Cancer Inst. 1999; 91: 1616–1634.CrossRef,PubMed,CAS,Web of Science® Times Cited: 34111
[99] Glaspy J. The impact of epoetin alfa on quality of life during cancer chemotherapy: a fresh look at an old problem. Semin Hematol. 1997; 34: 20–26.PubMed,CAS,Web of Science® Times Cited: 4112
[100] Jilani SM, Glaspy JA. Impact of epoetin alfa in chemotherapy-associated anemia. Semin Oncol. 1998; 25: 571–576.PubMed,CAS,Web of Science® Times Cited: 1621
[101] Dusenbery KE, McGuire WA, Holt PJ, et al. Erythropoietin increases hemoglobin during radiation therapy for cervical cancer. Int J Radiat Oncol Biol Phys. 1994; 29: 1079–1084.PubMed,CAS,Web of Science® Times Cited: 10128
[102] Wun T, Law L, Harvey D, Sieracki B, Scudder S et al. Increased Incidence of Symptomatic Venous Thrombosis in Patients with Cervical Carcinoma Treated

with Concurrent Chemotherapy, Radiation, and Erythropoietin. Cancer. 2003 Oct 1;98(7):1514-20.

[103] Bohlius J, Wilson J, Seidenfeld J, Piper M, Schwarzer G, Sandercock J, et al. Erythropoietin or darbepoetin for patients with cancer. Cochrane Database Syst Rev. 2006;3:CD003407. 10.1002/14651858.CD003407.pub4.

[104] Valles J, Santos MT, Aznar J, et al. Platelet-erythrocyte interactions enhance alpha(IIb)beta(3) integrin receptor activation and P-selectin expression during platelet recruitment: down-regulation by aspirin ex vivo. Blood. 2002; 99: 3978-3984.CrossRef,PubMed,CAS,Web of Science® Times Cited: 5635

[105] Valles J, Santos MT, Aznar J, et al. Erythrocyte promotion of platelet reactivity decreases the effectiveness of aspirin as an antithrombotic therapeutic modality: the effect of low-dose aspirin is less than optimal in patients with vascular disease due to prothrombotic effects of erythrocytes on platelet reactivity. Circulation. 1998; 97: 350–355.PubMed,CAS,Web of Science® Times Cited: 11236

[106] Santos MT, Valles J, Aznar J, Marcus AJ, Broekman MJ, Safier LB. Prothrombotic effects of erythrocytes on platelet reactivity. Reduction by aspirin. Circulation. 1997; 95: 63–68.PubMed,CAS,Web of Science® Times Cited: 8037

[107] Marcus AJ. Thrombosis and inflammation as multicellular processes: significance of cell-cell interactions. Semin Hematol. 1994; 31: 261–269.PubMed,CAS,Web of Science® Times Cited: 5638

[108] Valles J, Santos MT, Aznar J, et al. Erythrocytes metabolically enhance collagen-induced platelet responsiveness via increased thromboxane production, adenosine diphosphate release, and recruitment. Blood. 1991; 78: 154–162.PubMed,CAS,Web of Science® Times Cited: 12639

[109] Wun T, Paglieroni T, Hammond WP, Kaushansky K, Foster DC. Thrombopoietin is synergistic with other hematopoietic growth factors and physiologic platelet agonists for platelet activation in vitro. Am J Hematol. 1997; 54: 225–232.Direct Link:AbstractPDF(197K)References40

[110] Stohlawetz PJ, Dzirlo L, Hergovich N, et al. Effects of erythropoietin on platelet reactivity and thrombopoiesis in humans. Blood. 2000; 95: 2983-2989.PubMed,CAS,Web of Science® Times Cited: 9341

[111] Diaz-Ricart M, Etebanell E, Cases A, et al. Erythropoietin improves signaling through tyrosine phosphorylation in platelets from uremic patients. Thromb Haemost. 1999; 82: 1312–1317.PubMed,CAS,Web of Science® Times Cited: 2042

[112] Goel MS, Diamond SL. Adhesion of normal erythrocytes at depressed venous shear rates to activated neutrophils, activated platelets, and fibrin polymerized from plasma. Blood. 2002; 100: 3797–3803.CrossRef,PubMed,CAS,Web of Science® Times Cited: 27

[113] Barbui T, Finazzi G, Grassi A, Marchioli M. Thrombosis in cancer patients treated with hematopoietic growth factors. Thromb Haemost 1996;75:368- 71.

[114] Falanga A, Marchetti M, Evangelista V, Manarini S, Oldani S, Giovanelli S, et al. Neutrophil activation and hemostatic changes in healthy donors receiving granulocyte colonystimulating factor. Blood 1999;93(8):2506- 14.

[115] Agnelli G, Caprini JA. The prophylaxis of venous thrombosis in patients with cancer undergoing major abdominal surgery: emerging options. J Surg Oncol. 2007;96:265–72.

[116] Rasmussen MS, Jorgensen LN, Wille-Jorgensen P, et al. Prolonged prophylaxis with dalteparin to prevent late thromboembolic complications in patients undergoing major abdominal surgery: A multicenter randomized open-label study. J Thromb Haemost 2006;4(11):2384 90.

[117] Verso M, Agnelli G. Venous thromboembolism associated with long-term use of central venous catheters in cancer patients. J Clin Oncol 2003;21:3665–75.

[118] Tesselaar ME, Ouwerkek J, Nooy MA, et al. Risk factors for Catheter Related Thrombosis in Cancer Patients. Eur J Cancer 2004; 14:2553-2259.

[119] Verso M, Agnelli G, Bertoglio S, et al. Enoxaparin for the prevention of venous thromboembolism associated with central vein catheter: a double-blind, placebo-controlled, randomized study in cancer patients. J Clin Oncol 2005;23:4057–4062. [PubMed: 15767643]

[120] Mismetti P, Mille D, Laporte S, et al. Low-molecular-weight heparin (nadroparin) and very low doses of warfarin in the prevention of upper extremity thrombosis in cancer patients with indwelling longterm central venous catheters: a pilot randomized trial. Haematologica 2003;88:67–73. [PubMed:12551829]

[121] Niers TM, Di Nisio M, Klerk CP, Baarslag HJ, Buller HR, Biemond BJ. Prevention of catheter-related venous thrombosis with nadroparin in patients receiving chemotherapy for hematologic malignancies: a randomized, placebo-controlled study. J Thromb Haemost 2007;5:1878–1882. [PubMed: 17723127]

[122] Geerts WH, Pineo GF, Heit JA, et al. Prevention of venous thromboembolism: The seventh ACCP conference on antithrombotic and thrombolytic therapy. Chest 2004; 126(3 Suppl):338S 400S.

[123] Korones DN, Buzzard CJ, Asselin BL, Harris JP. Right atrial thrombi in children with cancer and indwelling catheters. J Pediatr 1996;128:841–6.

[124] Paut O, Kreitmann B, Silicani MA, et al. Successful treatment of fungal right atrial thrombosis complicating central venous catheterization in a critically ill child. Intensive Care Med 1992;18:375–6.

[125] Cohen GI, Klein AL, Chan KL, Stewart WJ, Salcedo EE. Transesophageal echocardiographic diagnosis of right-sided cardiac masses in patients with central lines. Am J Cardiol, 1992;70:925–9.

[126] Kroger K, Grutter R, Rudofsky G, Fink H, Niebel W. Followup after Port-a-Cath-induced thrombosis. J Clin Oncol 2002;20:2605–6.

[127] Cobos E, Dixon S, Keung YK. Prevention and management of central venous catheter thrombosis. Curr Opin Hematol 1998;5:355–9.

[128] Adamovich K, Tarnok A, Szauer E. Successful treatment of a right atrial thrombus secondary to central venous catheterization. Orv Hetil 1999;140:1467–70.

[129] Cesaro S, Paris M, Corro R, et al. Successful treatment of a catheter-related right atrial thrombosis with recombinant tissue plasminogen activator and heparin. Support Care Cancer 2002;10:253–5.

[130] Kingdon EJ, Holt SG, Davar J, et al. Atrial thrombus and central venous dialysis catheters. Am J Kidney Dis 2001; 38:631–9.

[131] Forauer AR, Bocchini TP, Lucas ED, Parker KR. Giant right atrial thrombus: a life-threatening complication of longterm central venous access catheters. J Vasc Interv Radiol 1998;9:519–20.

[132] Huraib S. Right atrial thrombus as a complication of subclavian vein catheterization—a case report. Angiology 1992; 43:439–42.

[133] Barrios CH, Zuke JE, Blaes B, Hirsch JD, Lyss AP. Evaluation of an implantable venous access system in a general oncology population. Oncology 1992;49:474–8.

[134] Kock HJ, Pietsch M, Krause U, Wilke H, Eigler FW. Implantable vascular access systems: experience in 1500 patients with totally implanted central venous port systems. World J Surg 1998;22:12–6.

[135] The Journal of Bone & Joint Surgery. Levels of Evidence for Primary Research Question, Instructions to Authors. Available at: http://www2.ejbjs.org/misc/instrux.shtml

[136] Lokich JJ, Bothe A Jr, Benotti P, Moore C. Complications and management of implanted venous access catheters. J Clin Oncol 1985;3:710–7.

[137] Ageno W, Huisman MV. Low-molecular-weight heparins in the treatment of venous thromboembolism. Curr Control Trials Cardiovasc Med 2000;1:102–5.

[138] Pucheu A, Dierhas M, Leduc B, et al. Fibrinolysis of deep venous thrombosis on implantable perfusion devices. Apropos of a consecutive series of 57 cases of thrombosis and 32 cases of fibrinolysis. Bull Cancer 1996;83:293–9.

[139] Schwarz RE, Groeger JS, Coit DG. Subcutaneously implanted central venous access devices in cancer patients: a prospective analysis. Cancer 1997;79:1635–40.

[140] Jacobs BR, Haygood M, Hingl J. Recombinant tissue plasminogen activator in the treatment of central venous catheter occlusion in children. J Pediatr 2001;139:593–6.

[141] Timoney JP, Malkin MG, Leone DM, et al. Safe and cost effective use of alteplase for the clearance of occluded central venous access devices. J Clin Oncol 2002;20:1918–22.

[142] Hooke C. Recombinant tissue plasminogen activator for central venous access device occlusion. J Pediatr Oncol Nurs 2000;17:174–8.

[143] Davis SN, Vermeulen L, Banton J, Schwartz BS, Williams EC. Activity and dosage of alteplase dilution for clearing occlusions of venous-access devices. Am J Health Syst Pharm 2000;57:1039–45.

[144] Food and Drug Administration. FDA Talk Paper: Serious Manufacturing eficiencies with Abbokinase Prompt FDA Letter to Abbott Labs. Rockville FL, MD: FDA. Available at: http://www.fda.gov/bbs/topics/ANSWERS/ ANS00964.html [Date accessed: July 16, 1999]

[145] Morris M, Eifel PJ, Lu J, et al. Pelvic radiation with concurrent chemotherapy compared with pelvic and para-aortic radiation for high-risk cervical cancer. N Engl J Med. 1999; 340: 1137–1143.

[146] Keys HM, Bundy BN, Stehman FB, et al. Cisplatin, radiation, and adjuvant hysterectomy compared with radiation and adjuvant hysterectomy for bulky Stage IB cervical carcinoma. N Engl J Med. 1999; 340: 1154–1161.

[147] Peters WA III, Liu PY, Barrett RJ, et al. Concurrent chemotherapy and pelvic radiation therapy compared with pelvic radiation therapy alone as adjuvant therapy after radical surgery in high-risk early-stage cancer of the cervix. J Clin Oncol. 2000; 18: 1606–1613.

[148] Whitney CW, Sause W, Bundy BN, et al. Randomized comparison of fluorouracil plus cisplatin versus hydroxyurea as an adjunct to radiation therapy in Stage IIB–IVA carcinoma of the cervix with negative para-aortic lymph nodes: a Gynecologic

Oncology Group and Southwest Oncology Group study. J Clin Oncol. 1999; 17: 1339–1348.

[149] Veronesi U, Maisonneuve P, Costa A, Sacchini V, Maltoni C, Robertson C, Rotmensz N, Boyle P. Prevention of breast cancer with tamoxifen: preliminary findings from the Italian randomised trial among hysterectomised women.Lancet. 1998; 352: 93–97.

[150] Cuzick J, Forbes J, Edwards R, Baum M, Cawthorn S, Coates A, Hamed A, Howell A, Powles T; IBIS investigators. First results from the International Breast Cancer Intervention Study (IBIS-I): a randomized prevention trial.Lancet. 2002; 360: 817–824.

[151] Fisher B, Costantino JP, Wickerham DL, Redmond CK, Kavanah M, Cronin WM, Vogel V, Robidoux A, Dimitrov N, Atkins J, Daly M, Wieand S, Tan-Chiu E, Ford L, Wolmark N. Tamoxifen for prevention of breast cancer: report of the National Surgical Adjuvant Breast and Bowel Project P-1 Study. J Natl Cancer Inst. 1998; 90: 1371–1388.

[152] Powles T, Eeles R, Ashley S, Easton D, Chang J, Dowsett M, Tidy A, Viggers J, Davey J. Interim analysis of the incidence of breast cancer in the Royal Marsden Hospital tamoxifen randomized chemoprevention trial. Lancet.1998; 352: 98–101.

[153] Cuzick J, Powles T, Veronesi U, Forbes J, Edwards R, Ashley S, Boyle P. Overview of the main outcomes in breast-cancer prevention trials. Lancet.2003; 361: 296–300.

[154] Tamoxifen for early breast cancer: an overview of the randomised trials. Early Breast Cancer Trialists' Collaborative Group. Lancet. 1998; 351: 1451–1467.

[155] Coombes RC, Hall E, Gibson LJ, Paridaens R, Jassem J, Delozier T, Jones SE, Alvarez I, Bertelli G, Ortmann O, Coates AS, Bajetta E, Dodwell D, Coleman RE, Fallowfield LJ, Mickiewicz E, Andersen J, Lonning PE, Cocconi G, Stewart A, Stuart N, Snowdon CF, Carpentieri M, Massimini G, Bliss JM; Intergroup Exemestane Study. A randomized trial of exemestane after two to three years of tamoxifen therapy in postmenopausal women with primary breast cancer.N Engl J Med. 2004; 350: 1081–1092.

[156] Prandoni P, Falanga A, Piccioli A. Cancer and venous thromboembolism. Lancet Oncol 2005; 6:401–410

[157] Heit JA, Silverstein MD, Mohr DN, Petterson TM, O'Fallon WM, Melton LJ 3rd. Risk factors for deep vein thrombosis and pulmonary embolism: a population-based case-control study. Arch Intern Med 2000; 160:809–815.

[158] Prins MH, Hettiarachchi RJ, Lensing AW, Hirsh J. Newly diagnosed malignancy in patients with venous thromboembolism: search or wait and see? Thromb Haemost 1997; 78:121–125

[159] Monreal M, Fernandez-Llamazares J, Perandreu J, Urrutia A, Sahuquillo JC, Contel E. Occult cancer in patients with venous thromboembolism:which patients, which cancers. Thromb Haemost 1997; 78:1316–1318

[160] Piccioli A, Prandoni P, Ewenstein BM, Goldhaber SZ. Cancer and venous thromboembolism. Am Heart J 1996; 132:850–855

[161] Piccioli A, Lensing AW, Prins MH, et al. Extensive screening for occult malignant disease in idiopathic venous thromboembolism: a prospective randomized clinical trial. J Thromb Haemost 2004; 2:884–889

[162] Rickles FR, Levine MN. Venous Thromboembolism in Malignancy and Malignancy in Venous Thromboembolism. Haemostasis 1998;28(Suppl.3):43-49.

[163] Nordström M, Lindblad B, Anderson H, Bergqvist D, Kjellström T. Deep venous thrombosis and occult malignancy: an epidemiological study. BMJ. 1994 April 2; 308(6933): 891–894.

[164] Lee AY. Thrombosis and cancer: the role of screening for occult cancer and recognizing the underlying biological mechanisms. Hematology Am Soc Hematol Educ Program 2006:438–443

[165] Budoff MJ, Fischer H, Gopal A. Incidental findings with cardiac CT evaluation: should we read beyond the heart? Catheter Cardiovasc Interv 2006; 68:965–973.

[166] Alikhan R, Cohen AT, Combe S, Samama MM, Desjardins L, Eldor A, et al. Prevention of venousthromboembolism in medical patients with enoxaparin: a subgroup analysis of the MEDENOX study. Blood Coag Fibrinolysis 2003;14:341–6.

[167] Bona RD, Hickey AD, Wallace DM. Efficacy and safety of oral anticoagulation in patients with cancer. Thromb Haemost 1997;78:137–140. [PubMed: 9198143]

[168] Khorana AA, Kuderer NM, Culakova E, Lyman GH, Francis CW. Development and validation of a predictive model for chemotherapy-associated thrombosis. Blood 2008;111:4902–7.

[169] Trujillo-Santos J, Di Micco P, Iannuzzo M, Lecumberri R, Guijarro R, Madridano O, Monreal M, and RIETE Investigators. Elevated white blood cell count and outcome in cancer patients with venous thromboembolism. Findings from the RIETE Registry. Thromb Haemost 2008;100:905–11.

[170] Falanga A, Levine MN, Consonni R, et al. The effect of very-low-dose warfarin on markers of hypercoagulation in metastatic breast cancer: Results from a randomized trial. Thromb Haemost 1998;79(1):23 7.

[171] ten Wolde M, Kraaijenhagen RA, Prins MH, Buller HR. The clinical usefulness of D-dimer testing in cancer patients with suspected deep venous thrombosis. Arch Intern Med. 2002;162:1880–4.

[172] Vormittag CR, Dunkler D, Simanek R, Chiriac AL, Drach J, Quehenberger P, Wagner O, Zielinski C, Pabinger I. D-dimer and prothrombin fragment 1 + 2 predict venous thromboembolism in patients with cancer: results from the Vienna Cancer and Thrombosis Study. J Clin Oncol 2009;27:4124–9.

[173] Uno K, Homma S, Satoh T, Nakanishi K, Abe D, Matsumoto K, et al. Tissue factor expression as a possible determinant of thromboembolism in ovarian cancer. Brit J Can 2007;96:290–5.

[174] Nemerson Y. Tissue factor and hemostasis. Blood 1988;71(1):1 8.

[175] Edgington TS, Mackman N, Brand K, et al. The structural biology of expression and function of tissue factor. Thromb Haemost 1991;66(1):67 79.

[176] Nakasaki T, Wada H, Shigemori C, et al. Expression of tissue factor and vascular endothelial growth factor is associated with angiogenesis in colorectal cancer. Am J Hematol 2002; 69(4):247 54.

[177] Poon RT, Lau CP, Ho JW, et al. Tissue factor expression correlates with tumor angiogenesis and invasiveness in human hepatocellular carcinoma. Clin Cancer Res 2003;9(14):5339 45.

[178] Ohta S, Wada H, Nakazaki T, et al. Expression of tissue factor is associated with clinical features and angiogenesis in prostate cancer. Anticancer Res 2002;22(5):2991 6.

[179] Leonardi MJ, McGory ML, Ko CY. A systematic review of deep venous thrombosis prophylaxis in cancer patients: implications for improving quality. Ann Surg Oncol 2007;14(2):929-36.

[180] Ay C, Simanek R, Vormittag R, Dunkler D, Alguel G, Koder S, Kornek G, Marosi C, Wagner O, Zielinski C, Pabinger I. High plasma levels of soluble P-selectin are predictive of venous thromboembolism in cancer patients - results from the Vienna Cancer and Thrombosis Study (CATS). Blood. 2008;112(7):2703-8.

[181] Kuenen BC, Levi M, Meijers JC, et al. Potential role of platelets in endothelial damage observed during treatment with cisplatin, gemcitabine, and the angiogenesis inhibitor SU5416. J Clin Oncol 2003;21(11):2192 8.

[182] Altinbas M, Coskun HS, Er O, et al. A randomized clinical trial of combination chemotherapy with and without low-molecular-weight heparin in small cell lung cancer. J Thromb Haemost 2004;2:1266–1271. [PubMed: 15304029]

[183] Lee AY, Rickles FR, Julian JA, et al. Randomized comparison of low molecular weight heparin and coumarin derivatives on the survival of patients with cancer and venous thromboembolism. J Clin Oncol 2005;23:2123–2129. [PubMed: 15699480]

[184] Barbui T, Falanga A. Disseminated intravascular coagulation in acute leukemia. Semin Thromb Hemost. 2001;27:593–604. [PubMed]

[185] De Stefano V, Sora F, Rossi E, et al. The risk of thrombosis in patients with acute leukemia: occurrence of thrombosis at diagnosis and during treatment. J Thromb Haemost. 2005;3:1985–1992. [PubMed]

[186] Ziegler S, Sperr WR, Knobl P, et al. Symptomatic venous thromboembolism in acute leukemia: incidence, risk factors, and impact on prognosis. Thromb Res. 2005;115:59–64. [PubMed]VTE in Central Nervous System Lymphoma.

[187] Quevedo JF, Buckner JC, Schmidt JL, et al. Thromboembolism in patients with high grade glioma. MayoClin Proc. 1994; 69: 329–332.

[188] Marras LC, Geerts WH, Perry JR. The risk of venous thromboembolism is increased throughout the course of malignant glioma. Cancer. 2000; 89: 640–646.

[189] Wen PY, Marks PW. Medical management of patients with brain tumors. Curr Opin Oncol. 2002; 14: 299–307.

[190] Walsh DC, Kakkar AK. Thromboembolism in brain tumors. Curr Opin Pulmonary Med. 2001; 7: 326-331.

[191] Clarke CS, Ortidge BW, Carney DN. Thromboembolism: a complication of weekly chemotherapy in the treatment of non-Hodgkin lymphoma. Cancer. 1990; 66: 2027–2030.

[192] Seifter EJ, Young RC, Longo DL. Deep venous thrombosis during therapy for Hodgkin's disease. Cancer Treat Rep. 1985; 69: 1011–1013.

[193] Genvresse I, Luftner D, Spath-Schwalbe E, Buttgereit F. Prevalence and clinical significance of anticardiolipin and anti-β2-glycoprotein-I antibodies in patients with non-Hodgkin's lymphoma. Eur J Haematol. 2002; 68: 84–90.

[194] Conlon SJ, White RH, Chew HK, Wun T. Incidence of Venous Thromboembolism in Patients wtih Lymphoma. J Thromb Haemost 2009;7(s2):168.

[195] Ku GH, White RH, Chew HK, Harvey DJ, Zhou H, Wun T. Venous thromboembolism in patients with acute leukemia: incidence, risk factors, and effect on survival. Blood 2009 Apr 23;113(17):3911-7

[196] Luong NV, Faderl S, Kantarjian H, Vu K. Prevalence of venous thromboembolism (VTE) among patients (pts) with acute leukemia (AL) prior to treatment. J Clin Oncol 29: 2011 (suppl; abstr 6595).

[197] Falanga A, Rickles F. Management of Thrombohemorrhagic Syndromes (THS) in Hematologic Malignancies. Hematology Am Soc Hematol Educ Program. 2007:165-71.

[198] Barbui T, FinazziG, Falanga A. The impact of all-trans-retinoic acid on the coagulopathy of acute promyelocytic leukemia. Blood 1998; 91: 3093–102.

[199] Runde V, Aul C, Heyll A, Schneider W. All-trans retinoic acid: not only a differentiating agent, but also an inducer of thromboembolic events in patients with M3 leukemia. Blood 1992; 79: 534–5.

[200] Musallam KM, Dahdaleh FS, Shamseddine AI, Taher AT. Incidence and prophylaxis of venous thromboembolic events in multiple myeloma patients receiving immunomodulatory therapy. Thromb Res. 2009 Mar;123(5):679-86. Epub 2008 Nov 6. Review.

[201] Sallah S, Hussain A, Wan J, Vos P, Nguyen NP. The risk of venous thromboembolic disease in patient with monoclonal gammopathy of undetermined significance. Ann Oncol. 2004;15:1490-1494. [Pubmed:17023574]

[202] Srkalovic G, Cameron MG, Rybicki L, Deitcher SR, Kattke-Merchant K, Hussein MA. Monoclonal gammopathy of undetermined significance and multiple myeloma are associated with an increased of venothromboembolic disease. Cancer.2004; 101:558-566.[PubMed:15274069]

[203] Kristinsson SY, Fears TR, Gridley G, Turesson I, Mellqvist UH, Bjorkholm M, et al. Deep vein thrombosis after monoclonal gammopathy of undetermined significance and multiple myeloma. Blood 2008 Nov 1;112(9):3582–6.

[204] Yang X, Brandenburg NA, Freeman J, Salomon ML, Zeldis JB, Knight RD, Bwire R. Venous Thromboembolism in Myelodysplastic Syndrome Patients Receiving Lenalidomide: Results from Postmarketing Surveillance and Data Mining Tecniques. Clin Drug Investig. 2009;29(3):161-71.

[205] De Stefano V, Za T, Rossi E, Vannucchi AM, Ruggeri M, Elli E, et al., GIMEMA CMD-Working Party(2008) Recurrent thrombosis in patients with polycythemia vera and essential thrombocythemia: incidence, risk factors, and effect of treatments. Haematologica 93(3):372–80.

[206] Landolfi R, Di Gennaro L. Pathophysiology of thrombosis in myeloproliferative neoplasms. Haematologica. 2011 Feb;96(2):183-6.

[207] Cella G, Marchetti M, Vianello F, Panova-Noeva M, Vignoli A, Russo L, et al.(2010) Nitric oxide derivatives and soluble plasma selectins in patients with myeloproliferative neoplasms. Thromb Haemost 104(1):151–6.

[208] Barbui T, Carobbio A, Finazzi G, Vannucchi AM, Barosi G, Antonioli E, et al.(2011) Inflammation and thrombosis in essential thrombocythemia and polycythemia vera: different role of C-reactive protein and Pentraxin 3. Haematologica 96(2):315–8.

[209] Khorana AA, Kuderer NM, Culakova E, Lyman GH, Francis CW. Development and validation of a predictive model for chemotherapy-associated thrombosis. Blood 2008;111(10):4902-4907

[210] Ay C, Dunkler D, Marosi C, Chiriac C, Vormittag R, Simanek R et al. Prediction of venous thromboembolism in cancer patients. Blood. 2010 Dec 9;116(24):5377-82.Epub 2010 Sep 9.

[211] Mismetti P, Laporte S, Darmon JY, Buchmuller A, Decousus H. Metaanalysis of low molecular weight heparin in the prevention of venous thromboembolism in general surgery. Br J Surg 2001;88(7):913- 30.

[212] A double-blind randomized multicentre trial with venographic assessment. ENOXACAN study group. Br J Surg 1997;84(8):1099 103.

[213] Levine M, Hirsh J, Gent M, Arnold A, Warr D, Falanga A, et al. Double-blind randomised trial of a very-low-dose warfarin for prevention of thromboembolism in stage IV breast cancer. Lancet 1994;343(8902):886- 9.

[214] Mclean Sarah, Ryan K, O'Donnell JS. Primary thromboprophylaxis in palliative care setting: a qualitative systemic review. Palliative Medicine 2010: 24(4):386-395.

[215] Geerts WH, Bergqvist D, Pineo GF, Heit JA, Samama CM, Lassen MR, et al. Prevention of venous thromboembolism: American College of Chest Physicians Evidence-Based Clinical Practice Guidelines (8th Edition). Chest 2008;133(6 Suppl):381S-453S

[216] Languasco A, Galante M, Marín J, Soler C, Lopez Saubidet C et al. Adherence to local guidelines for venous thromboprophylaxis: a cross-sectional study of medical inpatients in Argentina. Thrombosis Journal 2011, 9:18.

[217] Pengo V, Lensing AW, Prins MH, Marchiori A, Davidson BL, Tiozzo F, Albanese P, Biasiolo A, Pegoraro C, Iliceto S, Prandoni P (2004) Thromboembolic Pulmonary Hypertension Study Group. Incidence of chronic thromboembolic pulmonary hypertension after pulmonary embolism. N Engl J Med 350: 2257–2264

[218] Meyer G, Marjanovic Z, Valcke J, et al. Comparison of low-molecular-weight heparin and warfarin for the secondary prevention of venous thromboembolism in patients with cancer: a randomized controlled study. Arch Intern Med 2002; 162: 1729-1735.

[219] Deitcher SR, Kessler CM, Merli G, et al, ONCENOX Investigators. Secondary prevention of venous thromboembolic events in patients with active cancer: enoxaparin alone versus initial enoxaparin followed by warfarin for a 180-day period. Clin Appl Thromb Hemost 2006; 12: 389-396.

[220] Hull RD, Pineo GF, Brant RF, et al, for the LITE Trial Investigators. Long-term low-molecular-weight heparin versus usual care in proximal-vein thrombosis patients with cancer. Am J Med 2006; 119: 1062-1072.

[221] Akl EA, Barba M, Rohilla S, et al. Low-molecular-weight heparins are superior to vitamin k antagonists for the long term treatment of venous thromboembolism in patients with cancer: a Cochrane systematic review. J Exp Clin Cancer Res 2008; 27: 1-22.

5

Thrombosis Associated with Immunomodulatory Agents in Multiple Myeloma

Jose Ramon Gonzalez-Porras and María-Victoria Mateos
Hematology Department, Hospital Universitario de Salamanca and IBSAL, Salamanca
Spain

1. Introduction

Patients with multiple myeloma (MM) are increasingly at risk for thromboembolic events (TEEs), usually venous thromboembolism (VTE) [1]. The introduction of thalidomide and lenalidomide has clearly improved outcomes in MM patients but these immunomodulatory agents (IMiDs) are also associated with higher rates of TEEs [2]. The pathogenesis of thalidomide/lenalidomide-associated thrombosis is multifactorial and poorly understood. Patients with MM who are being treated with schemes including combinations of either thalidomide or lenalidomide plus other agents should receive some form of thrombosis prophylaxis [3]. This chapter discusses the incidence, pathogenic mechanisms, prophylaxis and treatment of thalidomide/lenalidomide-associated TEEs.

2. Multiple myeloma and thrombosis

The risk of developing venous thrombotic complications for patients with cancer is approximately five times that of the general population (0.5 *vs.* 0.1%) [4]. Multiple myeloma (MM), characterized by the malignant proliferation of clonal plasma cells, accounts for approximately 10% of hematologic malignancies and affects older individuals (median age, 70 years) [5]. Thromboembolic events are a key concern in clonal plasma cells disorders, such as monoclonal gammopathy of undetermined significance (MGUS) as well as in MM. The exact incidence of VTE in MGUS is difficult to determine since reported VTE rates probably vary according to the level of diagnostic vigilance. The underlying medical problems that prompted laboratory testing for monoclonal may also increase the risk of VTE. Srkalovic et al [1] noted an increased incidence of VTE among patients with MGUS. They reported that 7.5% (13 of 174 patients) of patients with MGUS developed VTE at a median of 4 months (range, 0–67 months) after diagnosis. The cumulative VTE rate was 16% after 8 years of follow-up. A medical history of VTE, family history of VTE, immobility, low serum albumin level and an increase in leukocyte count were found to be correlated with increased incidence of VTE in patients with MGUS. In another retrospective study (310 patients with MGUS) the incidence of VTE was 6.1% after a median follow-up of 44 months [6]. Univariate analysis showed that age ≥ 65 years, M protein ≥ 16 g/l and disease progression to symptom MM were the significant risk factors for VTE. A retrospective review of U.S. Veterans Affairs hospital records from 1980–1996 reported an incidence of VTE of 0.9, 3.1 and 8.7% in veterans without a plasma cell dyscrasia, diagnosed to have

MGUS, and MM, respectively [7]. The incidence of VTE in MM patients is difficult to estimate and varies from 3-10%. On the other hand, the recent introduction of the anti-myeloma therapy class called immunomodulatory drugs (IMiDs), substantially increased risk of VTE in multiple myeloma.

The exact pathogenesis of thrombosis in plasma cell dyscrasia is multifactorial and poorly understood. Prothrombotic coagulation abnormalities are found in patients with newly diagnosed multiple myeloma, including elevated levels of von Willebrand antigen factor, factor VIII and tissue factor, as well as decreased protein S and thrombosposndin [8]. Proinflammatory and angiogenic cytokines such as interleukin-6, tumor necrosis factor and vascular endothelial growth factor (VEGF) are elevated in MM and could activate the coagulation system [9]. A recently described mechanism of hypercoagulability in cancer patients, including MM patients, is acquired activated protein C resistance (APC-R). APC-R, in the absence of factor V Leiden mutation, was present in almost one-quarter of newly diagnosed myeloma patients and significantly increased the risk of VTE [10]. The possible production of auto-antibodies against protein C in these patients could explain the transient APC resistance phenotype. However, to date, we know of no single prothrombotic abnormality that can be used to predict which patients with plasma cell dyscrasia will develop VTE. Other risk factors of MM-associated thrombosis are involved, such as older age, immobility, prior or family history of VTE and the presence of other medical comorbidities, immobility due to pain and/or surgery, indwelling central venous catheters, extrinsic venous compression by plasmacytomas, and the presence of inherited factors such as factor V Leiden. However, the dominant risk factor for VTE in MM is the type of drug administered.

3. Thalidomide and thrombosis

Thalidomide is a glutamic acid derivative that exerts potent anti-angiogenic and immunomodulatory activity and has revolutionized clinical management of patients with myeloma. Thalidomide is effective in relapsed or refractory and newly diagnosed MM. However, from experience with myeloma patients, VTE has recently emerged as the single most important complication. The anti-myeloma effect is mediated by several mechanisms in myeloma cells directly as well as by the microenvironment [11]. Thalidomide induces G1 growth arrest/apoptosis by inhibiting NF-KB [12] and activating caspase. It inhibits adhesion of myeloma cells to bone marrow stromal cells, and inhibits secretion of cytokines (VEGF, [13], βFGF, [14-16], HGF, [17], TNFa, [18], IL-6, [19] and soluble IL-6 receptor (sIL-6R) [20]); up-regulate ICAM-1, [21] VCAM-1, IL-10, [22-23] and IL-12, [24]. Finally, it induces T cell and NK cell anti-myeloma immunity and inhibits angiogenesis [25].

The occurrence of VTE with the use of thalidomide was reported for the first time by Osman and Rajkumar in two independent phase 2 trials [31] in 2001. The combination of thalidomide (100–200 mg/day), doxorubicin (36 mg/m^2 on the first day of each 28-day cycle,) and dexamethasone (40 mg daily on days 1–4, 9–12, and 17–20 of each cycle) produced symptomatic deep venous thrombosis in four of the first 15 enrolled patients (27%) and the trial was therefore stopped. The other phase 2 trial combined thalidomide and dexamethasone for the treatment of patients with newly diagnosed myeloma at the Mayo Clinic. Seven percent (3/45) had thrombotic events. Cavo [32] and Rajkumar [33] in another two phase 3 trials confirmed the preliminary observations of increased incidence of VTE in newly diagnosed MM treated with thalidomide plus dexamethasone (16 and 17% of VTEs). (*table 1 below*).

Regimen	n	Status of disease	Incidence (%)
Thalidomide in monotherapy			
Barlogie, 2001 [26]	169	RR	< 2
Bennet, 2001 [27]	326	RR	4.6
Rajkumar, 2002 [28]	31	RR	3.4
Tosi, 2002 [29]	65	RR	1.5
Weber, 2002 [30]	28	ND	3
Thalidomide / Dexamethasone			
Cavo, 2004 [32]	71	ND	16
Rakjumar, 2006 [33]	103	ND	17
Palumbo, 2004 [34]	120	RR	2
Dimopoulos, 2001 [35]	44	RR	7
Thalidomide / Melphalan / Prednisone			
Palumbo, 2006 [36]	129	ND	20
Facon, 2007 [37]	125	ND	12
Thalidomide / Melphalan / Dexamethasone			
Dimopoulos 2006 [38]	50	ND	9
Thalidomide / Dexamethasone / CTX			
Sidra, 2006 [39]	62	ND / RR	3.2
García-Sanz, 2004 [40]	71	RR	7
Dimopoulos, 2004 [41]	53	RR	4
Kropff, 2003 [42]	60	RR	9
Moehler, 2003 [43]	56	RR	7
Thalidomide / Chemotherapy			
Baz, 2005 [44]	35	ND/RR	58
Zangari, 2004 [3]	87	ND	34
Zangari, 2002 [45]	232	RR	16
Barlogie, 2006 [46]	323	ND	34
Schutt, 2005 [47]	31	ND	26
Zervas, 2004 [48]	39	ND	10

RR: refractory / relapsed; ND: newly diagnosed.

Table 1. Incidence of thalidomide-associated venous thromboembolism without VTE prophylaxis

Similarly, when thalidomide was combined with melphalan and steroids, the incidence of VTE was 9-20% in newly diagnosed elderly patients [36-38]. In all of these studies, the major risk of thrombosis occurs early after initiation of the treatment, when the tumor load is maximal. Thus, this complication may be related to the release of thrombogenic factors from myeloma cells rather than to cumulative drug exposure [49].

A meta-analysis of studies of thalidomide in MM, which involved 3,322 patients, showed that patients receiving thalidomide were 2.1 times as likely to have a VTE event compared with those who were not receiving thalidomide ($p<0.01$). Those receiving thalidomide plus dexamethasone were 3.1 times as likely to have a VTE event ($p<0.01$), and those receiving thalidomide in addition to other chemotherapy agents were 1.5 times as likely to have a VTE event ($p<0.01$) [2].

The pathogenesis of thalidomide-associated thrombosis has not yet been established. Zangari et al. [10] tested for hypercoagulability in 62 newly diagnosed MMs, and found that DVT was more frequent in those patients with acquired APC resistance (36 *vs.* 15%, $p<0.04$). The pre-existing elevated factor VIII coagulant activity and von Willebrand factor antigen have also been related with thalidomide-associated thrombosis [50]. In an experimental model, Kausahal et al. demonstrated that the addition of thalidomide to uninjured arterial endothelium did not cause any appreciable change, whereas thalidomide added to adriamycin-injured (8–24 h) endothelial cells resulted in endothelial dysfunction by altering the expression of PAR-1 in injured endothelium [51].

Cases of VTE that began shortly after the initiation of treatment with recombinant human erythropoietin in patients who had been receiving thalidomide for some time have been reported [52]. However, another study found no apparent increased risk of thrombosis in 199 cases of myeloma given thalidomide with or without erythropoietin. Of the 49 patients receiving both drugs, 8.1% developed thrombosis compared with 9.3% of the 150 patients on thalidomide who did not receive erythropoietin [53].

The genetic susceptibility to developing a VTE in response to thalidomide therapy has been also evaluated. The lack of a strong association with genetic variations in the coagulation cascade, such as factor V Leiden or G20210A prothrombin mutation, suggests that VTE risk is mediated via alternative mechanisms. Johnson et al [54] identified 18 SNPs, using a custom-built molecular inversion probe (MIP)-based single nucleotide polymorphism (SNP) chip. There were two "response to stress" groups: a response to DNA damage group, including *CHEK1, XRCC5, LIG1, ERCC6, DCLRE1B* and *PARP1*, and a cytokine response group containing *NFKB1, TNFRSF17, IL12B* and *LEP*. A third apoptosis-related group with *CASP3, PPARD* and *NFKB1* was also found.

Interestingly, no thromboembolic events were observed in a group of 30 patients with relapsed MM treated with a bortezomib, melphalan, prednisone and thalidomide (VMPT) combination despite the absence of any anticoagulant prophylaxis [55]. A recent review of phase 3 trials of bortezomib- and/or IMiD-based therapy in frontline MM, together with other studies of novel combination regimens concluded that bortezomib-based regimens were typically associated with DVT/PE rates of ≤ 5%, similar to those seen with melphalan-prednisone and dexamethasone, whereas IMiD-based bortezomib-free regimens were generally associated with higher rates [56]. These results suggested the existence of a protective effect of coadministration of thalidomide or lenalidomide with bortezomib [57-58]. Zangari et al prospectively described *in vivo* effects of bortezomib from routine tests of blood coagulation and platelet function in treated MM patients. This pilot clinical trial showed *in vivo* that even a short exposure to bortezomib can affect platelet function. Platelet aggregation was reduced after bortezomib infusion with most of the commonly agonists used (ADP, epinephrine and ristocetin) on both days of treatment [59].

The majority of thrombotic events described in patients receiving treatment with thalidomide have been venous, but occasional arterial thrombotic events have also been reported [60-63]. In a prospective analysis of arterial thrombosis risk, the incidence of arterial thrombosis in patients with newly diagnosed MM treated with three cycles of thalidomide, doxorubicin and dexamethasone (TAD group) was 4.5%. However, the true incidence of arterial thrombosis could have been underestimated in the TAD group due to prophylactic use of LMWH. High factor VIII:C levels, possibly reflecting disease activity, could contribute to the risk of arterial thrombosis especially in patients with known cardiovascular risk factors [64].

4. Lenalidomide and thrombosis

Lenalidomide, a more potent immunomodulatory derivative of thalidomide, was designed to increase the anti-myeloma efficacy of thalidomide, while possibly reducing side effects like neuropathy and thrombosis. However, although neuropathy is not an important lenalidomide-related side effect, thrombosis continues to be one of the most important side effects, especially when lenalidomide is given in combination with dexamethasone or chemotherapy (*table* 2).

Regimen	n	Status of disease	Incidence (%)
Lenalidomide in monotherapy			
Richardson, 2009 [65]	222	RR	4
Lenalidomide / Dexamethasone			
Dimopoulos, 2007 [66]	176	RR	11.4
Weber, 2007 [67]	177	RR	14.7
Zonder, 2005 [68]	38	ND	75
Rajkumar 2010 [69]	223	ND	26
Lenalidomide / Dexamethasone Low Dose			
Rajkumar, 2010 [69]	222	ND	12
Lenalidomide / Dexamethasone / Bortezomib			
Richardson, 2010 [70]	66	ND	6

RR: refractory / relapsed; ND: newly diagnosed.

Table 2. Incidence of lenalidomide-associated venous thromboembolism without VTE prophylaxis

In two large phase 3 trials comparing lenalidomide plus dexamethasone to dexamethasone alone without mandated thromboprophylaxis in patients with RRMM, the incidences of VTE in the LD arm were 11.4 and 14.7%, compared with 4.6 and 3.4% in the DEX alone arm [66-67]. The incidence was even higher in patients with newly diagnosed MM (up to 75%) who were treated with lenalidomide plus dexamethasone [68]. In all these trials conducted in RR and newly diagnosed MM patients, dexamethasone was given at high dose (three pulses of 40 mg for 4 days, total amount per cycle: 480 mg). Interestingly, the rate of VTE was significantly lower when lenalidomide was combined with low-dose dexamethasone (40 mg weekly; total dose per cycle: 160mg) compared with high-dose (26 *vs.* 12%, p=0.0003) [69].

Similar to thalidomide, low rates of VTE have been reported in MM patients treated with lenalidomide in combination with bortezomib. In a phase 1/2 study of lenalidomide plus dexamethasone and bortezomib without thromboprophylaxis, thrombosis was rare (6% overall) [70].

The role of ESA and lenalidomide in thrombotic risk is controversial. An increased thrombotic risk has been observed in patients who received concomitant ESA with lenalidomide plus dexamethasone [71], although a third study showed no impact of ESA [72].

5. Pomalidomide and thrombosis

Pomalidomide (CC4047) is a new IMiD with high *in vitro* potency. In a phase 1 trial evaluating CC-4047 alone in 24 patients with RRMM, 4 (17%) developed a TEE during the first year of therapy [73]. Thromboprophylaxis was given in the phase 2 studies of pomalidomide and low-dose dexamethasone [74-78].

6. Prophylaxis of TEE-related IMiDs

Patients with MM being treated with IMiDs-based combinations should receive thromboprophylaxis [79-80]. There are data showing benefit of using low-molecular-weight heparin (LMWH), full-dose warfarin and daily aspirin in myeloma patients receiving IMiDs drugs [3, 44, 81]. However, fixed-dose warfarin (1 mg/d) was ineffective in reducing the VTE rate [3, 36]. Currently, outpatient VTE prophylaxis is recommended by the Italian Association of Medical Oncology, the National Comprehensive Cancer Network, the American Society of Clinical Oncology, the French National Federation of the League of Centers Against Cancer and the European Society of Medical Oncology only for medical oncology patients receiving highly thrombogenic thalidomide- or lenalidomide-based combination chemotherapy regimens [80].

The 2008 International Myeloma Working Group consensus statement on VTE prophylaxis in myeloma patients receiving thalidomide or lenalidomide [81], recommends a prophylaxis strategy according to a risk-assessment model. Individual risk factors for VTE associated with thalidomide and lenalidomide therapy include: advanced age, a history of VTE, an indwelling central venous catheter, comorbid conditions (e.g, infections, diabetes, cardiac disease, etc), current or recent immobilization, recent surgery and inherited thrombophilic abnormalities. Myeloma-related risk factors include diagnosis and hyperviscosity. Therapy-related risk factors include high-dose dexamethasone, doxorubicin or multiagent chemotherapy in combination with thalidomide or lenalidomide, but not with bortezomib. The panel recommends aspirin for patients with ≤1 risk factor for VTE. LMWH (equivalent to enoxaparin 40 mg per day) is recommended for those with two or more individual/myeloma-related risk factors. LMWH is also recommended for all patients receiving concurrent high-dose dexamethasone or doxorubicin. Full-dose warfarin targeting a therapeutic INR of 2-3 is an alternative to LMWH, although little has been published about this strategy (see *figure 1 below*).

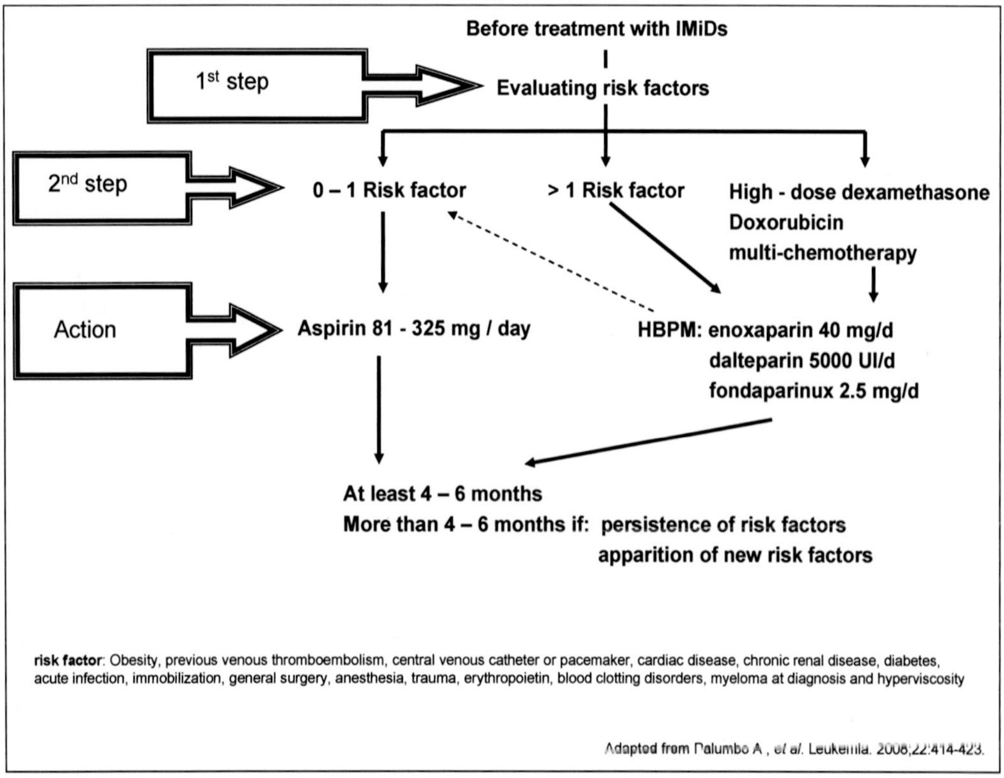

Fig. 1. International Myeloma Working Group consensus statement on VTE prophylaxis in myeloma patients receiving thalidomide or lenalidomide (2008).

Two direct comparison trials between thromboprophylaxis agents have recently been conducted. In the first phase 3 Italian Myeloma Network GIMEMA study [82], which prospectively assessed the impact of LMWH, aspirin or low-dose warfarin in newly diagnosed patients receiving thalidomide as part of either VMPT, VTD or TD regimens, the risk of VTE was similar in all three thromboprophylactic therapies after 6 months of follow up (5.0, 6.4 and 8.2%, respectively), and all were considered likely to be effective.

The second phase 3 trial compared the efficacy and safety of thromboprophylaxis with low-dose aspirin (ASA) or low-molecular-weight heparin (LMWH) in newly diagnosed MM patients, treated with lenalidomide and low-dose dexamethasone induction and melphalan-prednisone lenalidomide consolidation. The incidence of VTE was 2.27% in the ASA group and 1.20% in the LMWH group. The authors concluded that aspirin could be an effective and less expensive alternative to LMWH thromboprophylaxis during treatment with lenalidomide [83].

However, some questions remain unanswered: the outcome of the use of thromboprophylaxis in patients already in remission receiving thalidomide or lenalidomide as maintenance therapy during prolong periods of time is not well understood. A recent meta-analysis of the use of thalidomide as maintenance after autologous transplantation found the incidence of thromboembolic events to be 4–6%, and the risk of thromboembolism was 1.95 times that of patients who did not receive thalidomide [84]. The use of ASA for a longer period may reduce the risk of late thromboembolism. Future studies should address this possibility.

7. Management of IMiD-associated VTE

No studies or guidelines are available to guide treatment of established thalidomide/lenalidomide-associated VTE. Although the use of LMWH has improved VTE management in patients with solid tumors [85], no similar experience has been built up in patients with MM. The recommended treatment for thalidomide- or lenalidomide-associated thrombosis is either LMWH or warfarin. However, the use of LMWH is more attractive because of the lack of need for laboratory monitoring and the reduced variability (compared with warfarin) caused by interference from drugs and food. Also, in patients with solid tumors, LMWH administered for 6 months after a first VTE episode (1 month at full dose and 5 months at approximately 75% of the full dose) has proved to be safe and superior to warfarin in preventing VTE recurrence [85]. However, the optimal duration of anticoagulation therapy in oncology patients remains controversial.

The optimal doses of the most commonly used LMWH are 100 U/kg every 12 h or 200 U/kg daily for dalteparin, 1 mg/kg every 12 h or 1.5 mg/kg daily for enoxaparin, and 86 U/kg every 12 h or 171 U/kg daily for nadroparin. In patients with a high risk of hemorrhage (thrombocytopenia or renal failure), association of monitoring of peak anti-factor Xa levels to maintain a range of 0.5 to 1.0 IU/mL could be very attractive. In addition, a reduction of 50% of the therapeutic dose of LMWH for platelet counts less than 50 $x10^9/\mu L$, and a temporary discontinuation of LMWH for platelet counts less than 20,000 $x10^9/\mu L$ can be performed [86]. Also, UFH followed by warfarin remains a sensible alternative for VTE treatment in patients with CrCl <30 ml/min [87].

Zangari et al reported the treatment of 14 patients who developed thalidomide-related VTE. In 75% of them, administration of thalidomide was safely resumed after appropriate anticoagulation therapy was initiated. This consisted of low-molecular-weight heparin followed by warfarin, the target being the international normalized ratio of 2.5 to 3. Both anticoagulant and thalidomide treatments were continued as long as they were clinically indicated [88].

Alternative anti-myeloma treatment with an IMiS-free scheme should be seriously considered in patients who develop a VTE receiving LMWH or warfarin therapy with an appropriate INR [89]. However, if the use of IMiDs which produced the VTE is absolutely necessary, an alternative anticoagulant scheme could be used. In this setting, in patients with cancer-associated thrombosis while on warfarin therapy, with an appropriate INR, a recommended practice is to switch them to LMWH because it is more efficacious than warfarin [90]. On the other hand, dose escalation appears to be effective in patients who develop a cancer-associated thrombosis while on LMWH. In a small cohort study of oncology patients with recurrent thrombosis while on LMWH or warfarin, escalating the dose of LMWH by 20–25% or switching to LMWH, respectively, prevented further thrombotic episodes [91].

8. References

[1] Srkalovic G, Cameron MG, Rybicki L, et al. Monoclonal gammopathy of undetermined significance and multiple myeloma are associated with an increased incidence of venothromboembolic disease. Cancer. 2004;101: 558-566.

[2] El Accaoui RN, Shamseddeen WA, Taher AT: Thalidomide and thrombosis: A meta-analysis. Thromb Haemost. 2007;97: 1031-1036.

[3] Zangari M, Barlogie B, Anaissie E, et al. Deep vein thrombosis in patients with multiple myeloma treated with thalidomide and chemotherapy: effects of prophylactic and therapeutic anticoagulation. Br J Haematol. 2004;126: 715-721.

[4] Lee AY, Levine MN: Venous thromboembolism and cancer: Risks and outcomes. Circulation. 2003;107: I17-I21.

[5] Altekruse S, Kosary C, Krapcho M, et al. SEER Cancer Statistics Review 1975-2007. based on November 2009 SEER data submission, posted to the SEER website. http://seer.cancer.gov/csr/1975_2007/. Accessed 12 January 2011.

[6] Sallah S, Husain A, Wan J, et al. The risk of venous thromboembolic disease in patients with monoclonal gammopathy of undetermined significance. Ann Oncol. 2004; 15: 1490–1494.

[7] Kristinsson S, Fears T, Gridley G, et al. Deep vein thrombosis following monoclonal gammopathy of undetermined significance (MGUS) and multiple myeloma. Blood. 2008;112: 3582–3586.

[8] Auwerda JJA, Sonneveld P, de Maat MPM, et al. Prothromboic coagulation abnormalities in patients with newly diagnosed multiple myeloma. Haematologica 2007; 92: 279–280

[9] Fox EA, Kahn SR. The relationship between inflammation and venous thrombosis. A systematic review of clinical studies. Thromb Haemost. 2005;94: 362–365.

[10] Zangari M, Saghafifar F, Anaissie E, et al. Activated protein C resistance in the absence of factor V Leiden mutation is a common finding in multiple myeloma and is associated with an increased risk of thrombotic complications. Blood Coagul Fibrinolysis. 2002;13: 187-192.

[11] Hideshima T, Chauhan D, Shima Y, et al. Thalidomide and its analogs overcome drug resistance of human multiple myeloma cells to conventional therapy. Blood. 2000;96: 2943-2950.

[12] Keifer JA, Guttridge DC, Ashburner BP, et al. Inhibitor of NFKappa B activity by thalidomide through suppression of I Kappa B kinase activity. J Biol Chem. 2001;276: 22382–22387.

[13] Dankbar B, Padro T, Leo R, et al. Vascular endothelial growth factor and interleukin-6 in paracrine tumor-stromal cell interactions in multiple myeloma. Blood. 2000;95: 2630-2636

[14] Jakob C, Sterz J, Zavrski I, et al. Angiogenesis in multiple myeloma. Eur J Cancer. 2006;42:1581-1590.

[15] Sezer O, Jakob C, Eucker J, et al. Serum levels of the angiogenic cytokines basic fibroblast growth factor (bFGF), vascular endothelial growth factor (VEGF) and hepatocyte growth factor (HGF) in multiple myeloma. Eur J Haematol. 2001;66: 83-88.

[16] Urba ska-Rys H, Wierzbowska A, Robak T. Circulating angiogenic cytokines in multiple myeloma and related disorders. Eur Cytokine Netw. 2003;14: 40-51.

[17] Standal T, Abildgaard N, Fagerli UM, et al. HGF inhibits BMP-induced osteoblastogenesis: possible implications for the bone disease of multiple myeloma. Blood. 2007;109: 3024-3030.
[18] Hideshima T, Chauhan D, Schlossman R, et al. The role of tumor necrosis factor alpha in the pathophysiology of human multiple myeloma: therapeutic applications. Oncogene. 2001;20: 4519-4527.
[19] Klein B, Zhang XG, Lu ZY, et al. Bataille R. Interleukin- 6 in human multiple myeloma. Blood. 1995; 85: 863-872.
[20] Dmoszynska A, Podhorecka M, Manko J, et al. The influence of thalidomide therapy on cytokine secretion, immunophenotype, BCL-2 expression and microvessel density in patients with resistant or relapsed multiple myeloma. Neoplasma. 2005;52: 175-181.
[21] Geitz H, Handt S, Zwingenberger K. Thalidomide selectively modulates the density of cell surface molecules involved in the adhesion cascade. Immunopharmacology. 1996;31: 213-221.
[22] Gu ZJ, Costes V, Lu ZY, et al. Interleukin-10 is a growth factor for human myeloma cells by induction of an oncostatin M autocrine loop. Blood. 1996;88: 3972-3986.
[23] Lu ZY, Zhang XG, Rodriguez C, et al. Interleukin- 10 is a proliferation factor but not a differentiation factor for human myeloma cells. Blood. 1995;85: 2521-2527.
[24] Frassanito MA, Cusmai A, Dammacco F. Deregulated cytokine network and defective Th1 immune response in multiple myeloma. Clin Exp Immunol. 2001;125: 190-197.
[25] D'Amato RJ, Loughnan MS, Flynn E, et al. Thalidomide is an inhibitor of angiogenesis. Proc Natl Acad Sci USA. 1994;91: 4082- 4085.
[26] Barlogie B, Desikan R, Eddlemon P, et al. Extended survival in advanced and refractory multiple myeloma after single agent thalidomide: Identification of prognostic factors in a phase 2 study of 169 patients. Blood. 2001;98: 492–494.
[27] Bennett CL, Schumok GT, Kwaan HC, et al. High incidence of thalidomide-associated deep vein thrombosis and pulmonary emboli when chemotherapy is also administered (abstract). Blood. 2001;98: 863a.
[28] Rajkumar SV, Hayman S, Gertz MA, et al. Combination therapy with thalidomide plus dexamethasone for newly diagnosed myeloma. J Clin Oncol. 2002;20: 4319–4323.
[29] Tosi P, Zamagni E, Cellini C, et al. Salvage therapy with thalidomide in patients with advanced relapsed/refractory multiple myeloma. Haematologica. 2002;87: 408-414.
[30] Weber D, Ginsberg C, Walker P, et al. Correlation of thrombotic/embolic events (T/E) with features of hypercoagulability in previously untreated patients before and after treatment with thalidomide (T) or thalidomide-dexamethasone (TD) (abstract). Blood. 2002;100: 787.
[31] Osman K, Comenzo R, Rajkumar SV. Deep venous thrombosis and thalidomide therapy for multiple myeloma. N Engl J Med. 2001;344: 1951-1952.
[32] Cavo M, Zamagni E, Tosi P, et al: First-line therapy with thalidomide and dexamethasone in preparation for autologous stem cell transplantation for multiple myeloma. Haematologica. 2004;89: 826-831.
[33] Rajkumar SV, Blood E, Vesole D, et al: Phase III clinical trial of thalidomide plus dexamethasone compared with dexamethasone alone in newly diagnosed multiple myeloma: A clinical trial coordinated by the Eastern Cooperative Oncology Group. J Clin Oncol. 2006;24: 431-436.

[34] Palumbo A, Bertola A, Falco P, et al: Efficacy of low-dose thalidomide and dexamethasone as first salvage regimen in multiple myeloma. Hematol J. 2004;5: 318-324.

[35] Dimopoulos MA, Zervas K, Kouvatseas G, et al: Thalidomide and dexamethasone combination for refractory multiple myeloma. Ann Oncol. 2001;12: 991- 995.

[36] Palumbo A, Bringhen S, Caravita T, et al. Oral melphalan and prednisone chemotherapy plus thalidomide compared with melphalan and prednisone alone in elderly patients with multiple myeloma: randomised controlled trial. Lancet. 2006;367: 825-831

[37] Facon T, Mary JY, Hulin C, et al. Melphalan and prednisone plus thalidomide versus melphalan and prednisone alone or reduced-intensity autologous stem cell transplantation in elderly patients with multiple myeloma (IFM 99-06): a randomised trial. Lancet. 2007;370: 1209-1218

[38] Dimopoulos MA, Anagnostopoulos A, Terpos E, et al. Primary treatment with pulsed melphalan, dexamethasone and thalidomide for elderly symptomatic patients with multiple myeloma. Haematologica. 2006;91: 252-254.

[39] Sidra G, Williams CD, Russell NH, et al. Combination chemotherapy with cyclophosphamide, thalidomide and dexamethasone for patients with refractory, newly diagnosed or relapsed myeloma. Haematologica. 2006;91: 862-863.

[40] Garcia-Sanz R, Gonzalez-Porras JR, Hernandez JM, et al. The oral combination of thalidomide, cyclophosphamide and dexamethasone (ThaCyDex) is effective in relapsed/ refractory multiple myeloma. Leukemia 2004;18: 856-863.

[41] Dimopoulos MA, Hamilos G, Zomas A, et al. Pulsed cyclophosphamide, thalidomide and dexamethasone: an oral regimen for previously treated patients with multiple myeloma. Hematol J. 2004;5: 112-117.

[42] Kropff MH, Lang N, Bisping G, et al. Hyperfractionated cyclophosphamide in combination with pulsed dexamethasone and thalidomide (HyperCDT) in primary refractory or relapsed multiple myeloma. Br J Haematol. 2003;122: 607-616.

[43] Moehler TM, Neben K, Benner A, et al. Salvage therapy for multiple myeloma with thalidomide and CED chemotherapy. Blood. 2001;98: 3846-3848.

[44] Baz R, Li L, Kottke-Marchant K, et al. The role of aspirin in the prevention of thrombotic complications of thalidomide and anthracycline-based chemotherapy for multiple myeloma. Mayo Clin Proc. 2005;80: 1568-1574.

[45] Zangari M, Siegel E, Barlogie B, et al: Thrombogenic activity of doxorubicin in myeloma patients receiving thalidomide: Implications for therapy. Blood. 2002;100: 1168-1171.

[46] Barlogie B, Tricot G, Anaissie E, et al. Thalidomide and hematopoietic-cell transplantation for multiple myeloma. N Engl J Med. 2006;354: 1021-1030.

[47] Schutt P, Ebeling P, Buttkereit U, et al. Thalidomide in combination with vincristine, epirubicin and dexamethasone (VED) for previously untreated patients with multiple myeloma. Eur J Haematol. 2005;74: 40-46.

[48] Zervas K, Dimopoulos MA, Hatzicharissi E, et al. Primary treatment of multiple myeloma with thalidomide, vincristine, liposomal doxorubicin and dexamethasone (T-VAD doxil): a phase II multicenter study. Ann Oncol. 2004;15: 134-138.

[49] Anderson KC. Advances in disease biology: therapeutic implications. Semin Hematol. 2001;38(Suppl 3): 6–10.

[50] Ward CM, Yen T, Harvie R, et al. Elevated levels of factor VIII and von Willebrand factor after thalidomide treatment for malignancy: Relationship to thromboembolic events (abstract). Hematol J. 2003;4(suppl 1): 365.

[51] Kaushal V, Kaushal GP, Melkaveri SN, et al. Thalidomide protects endothelial cells from doxorubicin-induced apoptosis but alters cell morphology. J Thromb Haemost. 2004;2: 327-334.

[52] Steurer, M, Sudmeier, I, Stauder, R, et al. Thromboembolic events in patients with myelodysplastic syndrome receiving thalidomide in combination with darbepoietin-a. Br J Haematol. 2003;121: 101-103.

[53] Galli M, Elice F, Crippa C, et al. Recombinant human erythropoietin and the risk of thrombosis in patients receiving thalidomide for multiple myeloma. Haematologica. 2004;89: 1141–1142.

[54] Johnson DC, Corthals S, Ramos C, et al. Genetic associations with thalidomide mediated venous thrombotic events in myeloma identified using targeted genotyping. Blood. 2008;112: 4924-4934.

[55] Palumbo A, Ambrosini MT, Benevolo G, et al. Bortezomib, melphalan, prednisone, and thalidomide for relapsed multiple myeloma. The Italian Multiple Myeloma Network; Gruppo Italiano Malattie Ematologiche dell'Adulto. Blood. 2007;109: 2767-2772.

[56] Zangari M, Fink L, Zhan F, et al. Low venous thromboembolic risk with bortezomib in multiple myeloma and potential protective effect with thalidomide/lenalidomide-based therapy: review of data from phase 3 trials and studies of novel combination regimens. Clin Lymphoma Myeloma Leuk. 2011;11:228- 236.

[57] Ostrowska JD, Wojtukiewicz MZ, Chabielska E, et al. Proteasome inhibitor prevents experimental arterial thrombosis in renovascular hypertensive rats. Thromb Haemost 2004;92: 171-177.

[58] Wang M, Giralt S, Delasalle K, et al. Bortezomib in combination with thalidomide-dexamethasone for previously untreated multiple myeloma. Hematology. 2007;12: 235-239.

[59] Zangari M, Guerrero J, Cavallo F, et al. Hemostatic effects of bortezomib treatment in patients with relapsed or refractory multiple myeloma. Haematologica. 2008;93: 953-954.

[60] Goz M, Eren MN, Cakir O. Arterial trombosis and thalidomide. J Thromb Thrombolysis. 2008;25: 224-226.

[61] Altintas A, Ayyildiz O, Atay AE, et al. Thalidomide-associated arterial thrombosis: two case reports. Ann Acad Med Singapore. 2007;36: 304-306.

[62] Alkindi S, Dennison D, Pathare A. Arterial and venous thrombotic complications with thalidomide in multiple myeloma. Arch Med Res. 2008;39(2): 257-258.

[63] Raven W, Berghout A, van Houten A, et al. Treatment of multiple myeloma and arterial thrombosis. Ann Hematol. 2010;89(4):419–420.

[64] Libourel EJ, Sonneveld P, van der Holt B, et al. High incidence of arterial thrombosis in young patients treated for multiple myeloma: results of a prospective cohort study. Blood. 2010;116: 22-26.

[65] Richardson P, Jagannath S, Hussein M, et al. Safety and efficacy of single-agent lenalidomide in patients with relapsed and refractory multiple myeloma. Blood. 2009;114: 772-778.

[66] Dimopoulos M, Spencer A, Attal M, et al. Multiple Myeloma (010) Study Investigators. Lenalidomide plus dexamethasone for relapsed or refractory multiple myeloma. N Engl J Med. 2007;357: 2123-2132.
[67] Weber DM, Chen C, Niesvizky R, et al: Lenalidomide plus dexamethasone for relapsed multiple myeloma in North America. N Engl J Med. 2007; 357:2133-2142.
[68] Zonder JA, Durie BGM, McCoy J, et al. High incidence of thrombotic events observed in patients receiving lenalidomide (L) + dexamethasone (D) (LD) as first-line therapy for multiple myeloma (MM) without aspirin (ASA) prophylaxis (abstract). Blood. 2005;106:3455a.
[69] Rajkumar SV, Jacobus S, Callander NS, et al. Lenalidomide plus high-dose dexamethasone versus lenalidomide plus low-dose dexamethasone as initial therapy for newly diagnosed multiple myeloma: an open-label randomised controlled trial. Lancet Oncol. 2010;11: 29-37.
[70] Richardson PG, Weller E, Lonial S, et al. Lenalidomide, bortezomib, and dexamethasone combination therapy in patients with newly diagnosed multiple myeloma. Blood. 2010;116: 679-686.
[71] Niesvizky,R., Spencer,A., Wang,M. (2006) Increased risk of thrombosis with lenalidomide in combination with dexamethasone and erythropoietin (abstract). J Clin Oncol. 2006;24, 7506a.
[72] Menon SP, Rajkumar SV, Lacy M, et al. Thromboembolic events with lenalidomide-based therapy for multiple myeloma. Cancer. 2008;112: 1522-1528.
[73] Schey SA, Fields P, Bartlett JB, et al. Phase I study of an immunomodulatory thalidomide analog, CC-4047, in relapsed or refractory multiple myeloma. J Clin Oncol. 2004;22: 3269-3276.
[74] Lacy MQ, Hayman SR, Gertz MA, et al. Pomalidomide (CC4047) plus low-dose dexamethasone as therapy for relapsed multiple myeloma. J Clin Oncol 2009;27: 5008-5014.
[75] Lacy MQ, Hayman SR, Gertz MA, et al. Pomalidomide (CC4047) plus low dose dexamethasone (Pom/dex) is active and well tolerated in lenalidomide refractory multiple myeloma (MM). Leukemia. 2010;24: 1934-1939.
[76] Lacy MQ, Allred JB, Gertz MA, et al. Pomalidomide plus low-dose dexamethasone in myeloma refractory to both bortezomib and lenalidomide: comparison of two dosing strategies in dual-refractory disease. Blood. 2011;118: 2970-2975.
[77] Leleu X, Attal M, Moreau P, et al. Phase 2 study of 2 modalities of pomalidomide (CC4047) plus low-dose dexamethasone as therapy for relapsed multiple myeloma (abstract). Blood. 2010;116: 859a.
[78] Richardson PG, Siegel D, Baz R, et al. A phase 1/2 multi-center, randomized, open label dose escalation study to determine the maximum tolerated dose, safety, and efficacy of pomalidomide alone or in combination with low-dose dexamethasone in patients with relapsed and refractory multiple myeloma who have received prior treatment that includes lenalidomide and bortezomib (abstract). Blood. 2010;116: 864a.
[79] Palumbo A, Rajkumar SV, Dimopoulos MA, et al. Prevention of thalidomide- and lenalidomide-associated thrombosis in myeloma Leukemia. 2008;22: 414–423.

[80] Khorana AA, Streiff MB, Farge D, et al. Venous thromboembolism prophylaxis and treatment in cancer: a consensus statement of major guidelines panels and call to action. J Clin Oncol. 2009;27: 4919-4926.

[81] Palumbo A, Rus C, Zeldis JB, et al: Enoxaparin or aspirin for the prevention of recurrent thromboembolism in newly diagnosed myeloma patients treated with melphalan and prednisone plus thalidomide or lenalidomide. J Thromb Haemost. 2006;4: 1842-1845.

[82] Palumbo A, Cavo M, Bringhen S, et al. Aspirin, warfarin, or enoxaparin thromboprophylaxis in patients with multiple myeloma treated with thalidomide: a phase III, open-label, randomized trial. J Clin Oncol. 2011;29: 986–993.

[83] Larocca A, Cavallo F, Bringhen S, et al. Aspirin or enoxaparin thromboprophylaxis for newly-diagnosed multiple myeloma patients treated with lenalidomide. Blood. 2011[Epub ahead of print].

[84] Hicks LK, Haynes AE, Reece DE, et al: A meta-analysis and systematic review of thalidomide for patients with previously untreated multiple myeloma. Cancer Treat Rev. 2008;34: 442-452.

[85] Lee AY, Levine MN, Baker RI, et al: Low-molecular-weight heparin versus a coumarin for the prevention of recurrent venous thromboembolism in patients with cancer. N Engl J Med. 2003;349:146-153.

[86] Rickles FR, Falanga A, Montesinos P, et al. Bleeding and thrombosis in acute leukemia: what does the future of therapy look like? Thromb Res. 2007;120 Suppl 2: S99-106.

[87] Clark NP. Low-molecular-weight heparin use in the obese, elderly, and in renal insufficiency. Thromb Res. 2008;123 Suppl 1: S58-61.

[88] Zangari M, Anaissie E, Barlogie B, et al. Increased risk of deep-vein thrombosis in patients with multiple myeloma receiving thalidomide and chemotherapy. Blood 2001;98: 1614-1615.

[89] Zonder JA. Thrombotic Complications of Myeloma Therapy. Hematology Am Soc Hematol Educ Program. 2006;2010: 348-55.

[90] Lee AYY. Thrombosis in cancer: An update on prevention, treatment, and survival benefits of anticoagulants. Hematology Am Soc Hematol Educ Program. 2010;2010: 144-149.

[91] Carrier M, Le Gal G, Cho R, et al. Dose escalation of low molecular weight heparin to manage recurrent venous thromboembolic events despite systemic anticoagulation in cancer patients. J Thromb Haemost. 2009;7:760 - 765.

Section 3

Emerging Issues in Thromboprophylaxis

6

Aetiology of Deep Venous Thrombosis - Implications for Prophylaxis

Paul S. Agutter and P. Colm Malone
Theoretical Medicine and Biology Group, United Kingdom

1. Introduction

Clinical research on deep venous thrombosis (DVT) and thromboembolism (VTE) has focused in recent years on the contributions of potentiating factors, alone and in combination, to the risk of contracting these conditions. Many such 'risk factors' have been identified (Geerts *et al.*, 2004) and are discussed elsewhere in this book. The National Institute for Clinical Excellence (NICE) in the United Kingdom has exploited this knowledge to make the prevention of DVT its main focus for 2011. In his keynote lecture introducing the policy and procedures adopted by NICE, Arya (2011) described the tools for evaluating risk in various patient groups and emphasised 'anticoagulation' in the design and implementation of evidence-based prophylactic measures. He claimed that the frequency of VTE in hospital patients should be reduced by 2/3 if the agreed protocols are followed. An achievement of that magnitude would be most welcome.

Comparable views have been articulated elsewhere in Europe. Although NICE is distinctive in recommending assessment for thromboprophylaxis for all medical inpatients, the health services of other European Union countries offer broadly similar guidelines, especially for patients with acute medical conditions with expected durations of hospital stay longer than 3-4 days (Khoury *et al.*, 2011). Similarly, in the USA, the Surgeon General issued a 'Call to Action to Prevent Deep Venous Thrombosis and Pulmonary Embolism' in 2008 (Sliwka & Fang, 2010), and the Joint Commission on Accreditation of Healthcare Organizations requires prophylaxis for patients at moderate or high risk of VTE (Rothberg *et al.*, 2010). In all these cases, the emphasis is on anticoagulation, typically with unfractionated or low molecular weight heparin or with Fondaparinux.

However, despite the progress made in recent decades, the incidences of DVT-associated mortality and morbidity among hospital patients have declined only minimally (Kahn & Ginsberg, 2004; Heit, 2005), perhaps suggesting there is scope for improvement in our understanding of the aetiology of DVT and *a fortiori* our approach to prophylaxis.

Because of the range and variety of established risk factors, there is a widespread view that DVT is 'multifactorial' or 'multicausal' (e.g. Rosendaal, 1999, 2005; Lippi & Franchini, 2008; Khoury *et al.*, 2011). In a substantial minority of DVT patients, no known risk factor can be identified, and those cases are dubbed 'idiopathic'. While 'risk factors' determine the probability that a venous thrombus will become clinically significant and make embolism and/or post-thrombotic syndrome more likely, they have not been experimentally shown to be implicated in the *initiation* of thrombosis (Malone & Agutter, 2008, chapter 3). It is therefore conceivable that venous thrombogenesis *per se* is not multicausal.

The *valve cusp hypoxia* (VCH) *hypothesis* was proposed in the 1970s and was subsequently corroborated by experimental evidence showing that all cases of DVT have a common underlying aetiology (Malone & Agutter, 2006, 2008; Agutter & Malone, 2011). The (empirically validated) VCH thesis of DVT aetiology is rooted in longstanding causal concepts, but since it may be unfamiliar to some readers, it will be summarised in this chapter before we discuss its clinical implications. In section 2 the contrast between VCH and current mainstream views will be highlighted, and in section 3 we will explore its roots in the historical literature, focusing on Virchow's seminal studies of venous thrombi and emboli, which raised key questions that must be answered by a plausible account of their aetiology. Section 4 comprises an overview of the VCH thesis and its experimental validation, and answers those key questions. In section 5 the VCH thesis is extended in the light of recent publications, potentially enriching our understanding of DVT aetiology. Section 6 presents a rational approach to prophylaxis based on our understanding of VCH, and outlines a programme of experimental research leading to clinical trial/s.

2. A departure from mainstream views

The VCH thesis is rooted in and informed by the classical work of Virchow, Welch and Aschoff, and its account of DVT aetiology logically implies a means by which venous thrombogenesis can be anticipated and prevented; i.e. it provides a rational basis for prophylaxis, though not for therapy. The mainstream (consensus) viewpoint, in contrast, emphasises 'risk factors' to provide a basis for preventing or retarding the growth of already-formed thrombi. The two perspectives might therefore be seen as complementary rather than as necessarily conflicting, though they are very different.

For example, it is well established that inherited and acquired thrombophilias are important contributors to the risk for clinically significant DVT. After hereditary antithrombin III deficiency was described almost half a century ago (Egeberg, 1965) a number of thrombophilias were identified, and the molecular bases of many of them are now known. Defects in the protein C pathway are the most common inherited disorders (Lane *et al.*, 1996). Acquired thrombophilias are many and varied; the most widespread is antiphospholipid syndrome (Asherton & Hughes, 1989). There are many reviews of the field, e.g. Mazza (2004), Rosendaal (2005), Hassouna (2009), Anderson & Weitz (2010), and the topic is explored elsewhere in this book. Broadly, the work surveyed in these reviews shows that overactivity of coagulation factors, underactivity of regulatory factors or slow lysis of coagula can increase the risk of clinically significant DVT and embolism. Since a patient with no identifiable thrombophilia might develop DVT, it is supposed that other risk factors must be present to carry such patient over the presumed 'thrombogenic threshold' (Mammen, 1992; Lippi & Franchini, 2008; Anderson & Weitz, 2010).

According to the VCH thesis, however, thrombophilias do not *cause* DVT (Malone & Agutter, 2008, chapter 3). A thrombophilia increases the likelihood that a venous thrombus will become dangerous for the patient *after* it has formed, but it has no effect on the likelihood that thrombogenesis will occur in the first place. That does not diminish the relevance of thrombophilias to the *growth* of thrombi and *ipso facto* the likelihood of VTE, but it marginalises their significance for understanding aetiology and *a fortiori* for designing prophylactic measures. More generally: according to the VCH thesis, the situation or conditions under which venous thrombogenesis may be initiated, i.e. the *aetiology* of DVT, is not a defined haematological issue; no components of the coagulation mechanism are involved during the inception of the pathological process.

The introduction of haematological concepts and methods into the study of venous thrombosis is of quite recent origin. No haematological publication prior to the Second World War mentioned thrombosis (for example, see Eagle's excellent review 1938), and landmark studies of DVT made little or no reference to haematology. After 1945, considerations of haematology were only gradually introduced into the study of DVT (Robb-Smith, 1955); in the third edition of the Biggs-MacFarlane monograph on haematology (Biggs & MacFarlane, 1962), thrombosis was mentioned on only six of about 350 pages of text.

Virchow's seminal work (1856, 1858, 1862) was 'thrombological' not 'haematological', though this is a verbal rather than a clinical medical specification. Investigation of the haemophilia of Queen Victoria's child was already in hand as he organised his knowledge, but that investigation was wholly unrelated to his already-active studies of thrombosis and embolism.

3. Virchow's studies of thrombosis and embolism

Virchow's objective from 1846 to 1856 was to prove that pulmonary 'phlebitis' is actually 'pulmonary embolism' arising from thrombi formed in distal veins, and thus to contradict Cruveilhier. He wrote almost nothing of note about the mechanism(s) of thrombogenesis, but made crucial observations about the morphology of venous thrombi and the sites at which they form. Acceptable accounts of the aetiology of DVT must explain those observations.

Virchow's work on thrombosis and embolism has been widely misunderstood and misrepresented during the past half century.

3.1 The status and provenance of 'Virchow's triad'

In a generally excellent review, Bovill & van der Vliet (2011) wrote: "In the mid-nineteenth century, Rudolph Virchow described, in a paper on PE, three factors that he felt contributed to thrombogenesis (32). The three factors were blood flow (stasis or impaired flow), composition of the blood (hypercoagulability), and changes in the vessel wall (endothelial activation and or damage). This triad has guided thinking about thrombogenesis for 150 years." Their reference (32) is to a secondary source (Owen, 2001). The quoted passage from Bovill & van der Vliet sums up a common but mistaken belief about Virchow's contribution to the field (e.g. Peterson, 1986; Rosendaal, 2005; Esmon, 2009; Kyrle & Eichinger, 2009; Meetoo, 2010). Virchow wrote no such thing.

In both *Thrombose und Embolie* (Virchow, 1856) and the relevant lectures in *Die Cellularpathologie in ihrer Begründung auf physiologische und pathologische Gewebelehre* (Virchow, 1858), the focus was on pulmonary embolism, not thrombogenesis. The only passage in *Thrombose und Embolie* that vaguely resembles 'Virchow's triad' (pp. 293-4 of the Matzdorff-Bell translation) states: "*the sequence of the possible stages and consequences of blockage may be classified and studied under three headings: (1) phenomena associated with irritation of the vessel and its vicinity; (2) phenomena of blood-coagulation; and (3) phenomena of interrupted blood-flow*". But as the context makes clear, this refers to the 'blockage' of the pulmonary artery by a metastasised thrombus, not to the formation of that thrombus in a distal vein. The quoted passage from Virchow's classic appears to have been misread and mistranslated during the mid-20th century, perhaps because English-speaking readers found 19th century technical German difficult; there was no full and authoritative English translation of *Thrombose und Embolie* until 1998. Several authors have made this point (Brinkhous, 1969; Brotman *et al.*, 2004; Dickson, 2004; Malone & Agutter, 2006; Bagot & Arya, 2008), but the misinterpretation persists. Some of these authors claim that although 'Virchow's triad' has no basis in what Virchow wrote, it is nevertheless useful in clinical practice (Brotman *et al.*, 2004; Bagot & Arya, 2008). That may seem practical, guiding us to deal with injured veins, administer anticoagulants, and maintain a reasonably high venous blood flow rate in the lower limbs; but it is not scientifically honourable to exonerate and even legitimate an accidental and regrettable distortion of Virchow's meticulous observations to the detriment of our understanding of the aetiology of DVT.

The truth is that Virchow neither conceived nor wrote 'Virchow's triad'; the phrase first appeared in print following the historical study by Anning (1957), about a century after Virchow's seminal works were published.

3.1.1 Precedents and mutations of 'Virchow's triad'

In its original form - the statement that DVT is caused by some combination of disturbed blood flow, altered blood composition and vessel wall abnormality - 'Virchow's triad' was unexceptionable though misconceived. It afforded a general view of causation, and it is hard to imagine any contribution to the aetiology other than the three named facets. Moreover, it was one of a line of general points of view about DVT dating from the late 19th and early 20th centuries and thus belonged to an institutionalised tradition. For example, Aschoff (1924) proposed a 'tetrad': that DVT is caused by some combination of changes in the coagulability of the blood, changes in the formed elements of the blood, changes in the circulatory blood flow and changes in the vessel walls. But Virchow did not contribute to that tradition.

However, 'Virchow's triad' underwent mutations early in its history (late 1950s). 'Disturbed blood flow' came to be equated with 'venous stasis' (and to mean slow-flow rather than literally no-flow), just as 'altered blood composition' came to be interpreted as 'hypercoagulability'. It must be emphasised that Virchow never mentioned 'hypercoagulability' and furthermore explicitly rejected the 'doctrine' (*die Lehre*) that stasis has any causal role in thrombosis or embolism. 'Virchow's triad' would have bewildered him. The mutations continued and some authors, contrary to the superb studies by Welch (1887, 1899), have doubted whether vessel injury is causally significant in venous thrombosis (Comerota *et al.*, 1985; Kyrle & Eichinger, 2009); however, others such as López & Chen (2009) have recognised that events at the vessel wall precede coagulation. Moreover, retarded blood flow or 'stasis' is sometimes viewed as only a 'potentiating influence' because – so it is conjectured - it allows coagulation factors to accumulate locally (Thomas, 1988; Mammen, 1992; Hamby, 2005). Thus, increasing emphasis has been placed on the presumption of abnormally rapid blood coagulation (Thiangarajan, 2002; Bulger *et al.*, 2004), i.e. on thrombophilias, fostering the misleading impression that the aetiology of DVT is to be understood within the domain of haematology rather than that of circulatory anatomy and physiology.

Interestingly, the invention of 'Virchow's triad' in the late 1950s - and the concomitant assumption that DVT is a haematological disorder - followed in the wake of the FDA's acceptance of anticoagulant therapy and prophylaxis (Cundiff *et al.*, 2010). Some connection might be suspected, and was indeed suspected at the time. We have quoted the barbed comments of Pulvertaft (1947) elsewhere (Malone & Agutter, 2008). Robb-Smith (1955) wrote: "*In recent years haematologists have been forced to take an interest in the practical if not the theoretical aspects of thrombosis by the introduction of anticoagulant therapy.*" Later in the same article, he observed: "*… the coagulationist, tilting his tubes with stop-watch in hand, appears to have inherited the mantle of druidical haematomancy, like the medieval physician who based his prognosis on the appearance of the buffy coat in the bleeding bowl… one has the feeling that the stock-in-trade of reagents and reactions to produce a fibrin clot is remote from a thrombus*". Robb-Smith understood the spirit of Virchow's work. (Of course, he did not use the phrase 'Virchow's triad', which would not be coined for another two years.)

3.2 Virchow's *real* triad

Although Virchow's studies during the decade 1846-56 were motivated by refutation of Cruveilhier's opinions and therefore focused on the causation of pulmonary emboli, not of thrombosis, his observations of venous thrombi were crucially important, thanks to his skilled use of the Lister microscope (invented in 1827). One of these observations was his three-part contrast between a thrombus and an *ex vivo* clot. On pp. 514-5 of the *Gesammelte Abhandlungen* (Virchow, 1862), he recognised that:

1. a thrombus, unlike a clot, has a manifestly layered structure, later called the Lines of Zahn (Zahn, 1876);
2. the fibrin content is many times denser than is found in a clot;
3. the white cell content is vastly greater.

This tripartite distinction between 'venous thrombus' and 'clot' has a better claim to be labelled 'Virchow's triad' than the stasis-hypercoagulability-injury mantra, since Virchow actually wrote it. Moreover, it encapsulates common clinical knowledge; for instance, those who have seen a thrombus extracted during a venectomy or an embolism removed at post-mortem have had the opportunity to observe the white 'tail' (the *Kopfteil* in the terminology of Aschoff, 1924).

In view of the clarity of Virchow's summary distinction, the now-commonplace tendency to treat 'venous thrombus' as synonymous with 'clot' is surprising. Perhaps we should recall the elementary fact reported by Joseph Lister in his Croonian lecture (Lister, 1863): circulating blood has no inherent tendency to coagulate; coagulation is initiated *only* when blood makes contact with an abnormal surface, i.e. anything other than normal, uninjured vascular endothelium. Haemostasis is a part of normal physiology, initiated when blood leaks from a vessel. Venous thrombogenesis is not normal physiology; it is a pathological process entailing local blood coagulation *in situ*. A venous thrombus is a lesion, in the strict sense of an abnormal change in a tissue caused by injury or disease. Venous thrombi are in many respects *like* clots, but they are not clots, so it is not logical to infer that they are formed in the same way as clots.

3.2.1 The importance of Virchow's *real* triad

The morphological characterization of venous thrombi encapsulated in Virchow's publication is important in two respects:

First, an account of the aetiology of DVT must include a causal explanation for all three morphological features. That is the critical test of any aetiological hypothesis.

Second, Virchow's *real* triad constitutes a triple criterion for assessing experimental thrombi. Any coagulum or other structure produced in an experimental setting that does not display Lines of Zahn, dense fibrin and a white *Kopfteil* cannot be regarded as a thrombus, and the experimental model that generates such a structure cannot be considered a model for venous thrombogenesis (cf. Welch, 1887, 1899).

3.2.2 Leukocytes and venous thrombogenesis

Nowadays, notwithstanding Virchow's observations, it seems to be tacitly assumed that leukocytes have no aetiological significance and are concentrated in the *Kopfteil* of a thrombus only because they are adventitiously trapped in the fibrin mesh. But adventitious trapping cannot explain the segregated whiteness of the *Kopfteil*; erythrocytes are also adventitiously trapped by the fibrin and they outnumber leukocytes in the circulating blood by many orders of magnitude, hence the redness of the subsequent, more newly-formed, *Schwansteil* of a thrombus.

Virchow's key insight was that the leukocytes concentrated in a venous thrombus (as distinct from a clot) originate from within the blood stream, not from outside (migrating through the vessel wall) as previously supposed. *A fortiori*, they must form while the blood is *flowing*, since such an excess of leukocytes over erythrocytes can be provided only from a large volume of circulating blood. However, he was not the first investigator to recognise that white material is a primary constituent of what we now call 'venous thrombi'. Hunter (1793) wrote about the 'inflammation of the internal coats of veins', describing a lesion of the kind we now call 'venous thrombosis' as a local accumulation of 'pus'. Similarly, Cruveilhier focused on the accumulation of 'inflammatory' material, denoting the process by the term 'phlebitis' (Talbott, 1970). Unlike Hunter and Cruveilhier, who denounced the 'magnifying glasses' of their day, Virchow used the microscope, so he was able to see that the white material in a venous thrombus was not amorphous but comprised a mass of cells. Two decades later, the improved Zeiss microscope made platelets readily visible as obviously copious blood elements.

This observation inspired investigations of venous thrombi over the following seventy years. The elegant and detailed morphological studies of Welch (1887, 1899) highlighted the contributions of leukocytes as well as platelets to thrombus structure, and Aschoff (1924) declared that the causation of DVT would only be understood when the accumulation of white cells was explained: "*Along with the explanation of this marking* [the Lines of Zahn] *stands or falls the whole problem of thrombus formation, so far as consideration of the majority of cases of autochthonous thrombosis goes*".

3.2.3 Why do leukocytes accumulate at sites of venous thrombogenesis?

Hunter realised in 1793, more than 60 years before the germ theory of disease was articulated, that leukocytes swarm to sites of either tissue injury or local infection (a phenomenon more recently termed 'margination of leukocytes'). After Pasteur's work had been accepted, it was widely supposed that infections contribute to the causation of DVT; but when no consistent correlation between thrombosis and infectious agents was established, and antibiotics did not alleviate or prevent DVT, that hypothesis was abandoned during the first half of the 20th century. This aspect of history was reviewed briefly in our monograph (Malone & Agutter, 2008, chapter 7). Once again, Virchow was uncannily prescient on this topic; although unaware of the epoch-making discoveries being made in Pasteur's laboratory while he was writing *Thrombose und Embolie,* he perceptively described the accumulation of white material in thrombi as '*puriform but not purulent*' (Virchow, 1856).

For more than a century there has been experimental support for the inference that the cause of leukocyte and platelet margination at the site of venous thrombogenesis is local injury. Welch (1887, 1899) showed that experimental thrombi induced by electrical or other traumatic injury to the venous endothelium morphologically resembled autochthonous thrombi. This established the only valid way of evaluating experimental thrombi; as stated in section 3.2.1, coagula that lack the structure summarised in Virchow's *real* triad are not 'thrombi'.

The studies of Sandison (1931) and Stewart *et al.* (1974) supported Welch's conclusion: vessel injury (by whatever agency) causes the generation of thrombi indistinguishable from autochthonous ones - dominated by the accumulation of vast numbers of sequestrated/marginated white cells.

However, in most DVT cases encountered clinically and viewed microscopically, the venous endothelium appears ostensibly intact. Therefore, the key questions arising from the studies of Virchow and others (notably Welch and Aschoff) are: what causes the putative *subtle* injury to the venous endothelium that could initiate autochthonous thrombogenesis, and is a particular zone or area of venous endothelium involved?

3.2.4 A caveat

These two questions were the points of departure for the VCH hypothesis and their answers are fundamental to the VCH mechanism. However, Virchow's *real* triad does not only concern leukocyte/platelet margination at the site of thrombus formation. Its other two microscopic facets should not be overlooked: the remarkably high density of fibrin in those parts of a thrombus that are formed first, in the *Kopfteil;* and the extraordinary morphology of the Lines of Zahn. These observations remind us that despite the importance of leukocytes in thrombogenesis, their swarming around the site coincides with, and is often preceded by, local coagulation. In the tenth lecture in *Die Cellularpathologie,* Virchow (1858) overtly attacked Cruveilhier but made this exception: *"Cruveilhier was right... that the so-called pus in the veins never, in the first instance, lies against the wall of the vein, but is always seen first in the centre of a previously existing coagulum which marks the start of the process".*

This observation indicates that the subtle endothelial injury inducing local leukocyte/platelet swarming and margination also initiates local coagulation, which may proceed rapidly. But though Virchow did not speculate about the cause or nature of that subtle injury, he did pin-point its location.

3.3 Thrombi are formed in venous valves

Virchow (1856, 1858) showed that venous thrombi are formed in the valves, including the (usually monocuspid) valves that control vein junctions, which Franklin (1937) termed 'ostial valves'. The formation of thrombi in valves was mentioned in *Thrombose und Embolie* and two thrombi arising from two ostial valves were illustrated in *Die Cellularpathologie.* It is worth recalling that even the smallest veins have valves (Phillips *et al.*, 2004), which *ipso facto* are potential sites of thrombogenesis.

Although Virchow was the first investigator to make the critical role of valves in venous thrombosis explicit, thanks to his use of the microscope, both Hunter and Cruveilhier had probably suspected the same thing. Hunter (1793) was explicit in associating the 'inflammation' ('pus accumulation', i.e. thrombogenesis) with the 'internal coats' of veins, but he too was surprised that the structures he observed were formed in mid-lumen, not on the walls. Likewise, Cruveilhier was puzzled by the formation of 'phlebitis' in mid-lumen. Both these antecedents of Virchow held now-defunct views about what they were looking at: they believed that the 'pus' originated from outside the vessel, which made the observation of a notably centralised coagulum especially difficult to explain in contemporaneous terms. Hunter did not state explicitly that thrombi are initiated on the valves. He considered the microscope an unreliable instrument in his day and eschewed its use, and without the microscope it was/is impossible to see a valve smothered by a large thrombus. However, he was familiar with Harvey's (1628) essay on the circulation of the blood, in which the valves were described as *'eminences'* on the *'internal lining (tunicula intima)'* of the vein. Hence, we suggest, the title of Hunter's treatise (*'inflammation of the internal coats...'*) suggests that he, Cruveilhier and Virchow had observed that venous thrombi are 'anchored' - and probably initiated - on/in valve pockets.

A number of detailed studies during the third quarter of the 20th century confirmed Virchow's observation that thrombi are formed in venous valves (e.g. McLachlin & Paterson, 1951; Sevitt, 1974). One of us (PCM) inherited many micrographs of venous thrombi from Simon Sevitt after his death, some of which we used to illustrate our monograph (Malone & Agutter, 2008; see especially the photographs in Fig. 10.5). All his micrographs showed thrombi seated in the valve pockets. In some, the exact site of attachment to the endothelium is not clear because the entire pocket is filled with the thrombus, but in several images the thrombus is evidently attached to the inner (parietalis) face of the valve cusp leaflet, not to the outer (luminalis) face, and not to the vein wall. This recurrent observation played a crucial part in the formulation of the VCH hypothesis.

Bovill & van der Vliet (2011), examining the small sample of micrographs in Sevitt (1974), inferred instead that the thrombi were attached to the vein wall endothelium within the valve pocket. We shall discuss this divergence of opinion later; but it seems improbable that a thrombus perceived as 'anchored' in mid-lumen could be attached to the vein wall endothelium.

4. Valve Cusp Hypoxia: The basis of venous thrombogenesis

The foregoing background led us to articulate the VCH hypothesis and subsequently to validate it.

4.1 What severely embarrasses or kills the endothelium in a venous valve pocket?

The clue to what injures the endothelial lining of an intact, functioning, vein was suggested by Drinker (1938) and van Ottingen (1941), whose researches unexpectedly established that copious and ubiquitous thrombus-like coagula formed in the veins of the victims of carbon monoxide poisoning and were associated with endothelial alterations. Evidently, either carboxyhaemoglobinaemia or hypoxaemia could cause the endothelial injury associated with DVT. Drinker proposed this hypothesis to O'Neill (1947) who provisionally validated it, and Samuels & Webster (1952) supported the proposal. Malone & Morris (1978) showed that lesions similar to the white parts of autochthonous and experimental thrombi formed in the veins of oxygen-starved animals by the process of margination and sequestration of platelets and leukocytes. Interestingly, Samuels & Webster (1952) showed that heparin does not prevent the development of a nascent thrombus on a hypoxically injured endothelium.

In those mid-20th century papers, it was debated whether oxygen was supplied to the venous endothelium from the luminal blood or the vasa venarum. Presumably, hypoxia sufficiently severe to kill the endothelial cells and induce leukocyte swarming and phagocytosis of the debris required impaired oxygenation from both sources; it is well established that the venous endothelium can survive moderately prolonged hypoxia (Jackson *et al.*, 1988), depending on anaerobic glycolysis to provide ATP (Berna *et al.*, 2001), and surgeons procure the use of a bloodless field under a 2.5 hour tourniquet. However, hypoxia that is not so severe as to kill the cells but is sufficient to alter their phenotype can also lead to leukocyte and platelet recruitment and local coagulation. During the period 1980-2000, studies in a number of laboratories established that significant but non-fatal hypoxia in cultured venous endothelial cells induces the expression of the early growth response-1 (egr-1) gene, and this unleashes a cascade of gene-expression and phenotypic changes that would promote local coagulation and leukocyte accumulation *in vivo* (Pinsky *et al.*, 1995; Yan *et al.*, 1999a,b; Karimova & Pinsky, 2001; Ten & Pinsky, 2002).

4.1.1 The vagaries of 'venous stasis'

By the late 19th century it was clear that paralyzed patients develop DVT and PE (Malpother, 1880), and by the middle of the 20th century it was known that prolonged bed rest, e.g. in spinal injury patients, had the same consequence (Wright & Osborn, 1952; Gibbs, 1957). This association between restricted mobility and DVT was attributed to slowed venous return, i.e. reduced volume per unit time (Ochsner *et al.*, 1951; Wright & Osborn, 1952). Thus, by the early 1960s, it was held to be virtually certain that 'venous stasis' contributed to the cause of DVT (Zweifach, 1963); it was imagined to promote local coagulation (Mammen, 1992). The endothelial hypoxia hypothesis (from which the VCH hypothesis was coined) directly supported this premise: if blood were to flow slowly enough to injure some part of the endothelium by hypoxaemia (even to kill that part of the tissue should flow cease altogether in an unflapped, unemptied valve pocket), local leukocyte swarming and margination, and local coagulation, would ensue through the molecular mechanisms discovered by Pinsky and his colleagues.

However, that conception seems hard to reconcile with Hewson's (1771) experiment. Hewson doubly-ligated a dog's jugular vein, and the stationary blood between the ligatures failed to coagulate after more than an hour; even after three hours, coagulation was only partial. His finding was so counter-intuitive that Lister (1863) and Baumgarten (1876) repeated it in the 19th century and Wessler (1962) in the 20th, with identical results.

Wessler's findings indicated that double ligation *did* somehow injure the vessel, directly or indirectly, because rapid coagulation followed when he introduced serum containing activated coagulation factors into the ligated portion. Importantly, however, the resulting coagula bore no morphological resemblance to autochthonous venous thrombi, so – as explained in section 3.2.1 – his world-renowned experiments were of limited relevance for understanding the aetiology of DVT.

4.1.2 Resolving the 'stasis' paradox

Wessler's studies suggested what seemed like a paradoxical conclusion: thrombi can form when blood is flowing (albeit slowly) along a vessel segment, but not when the blood is stationary. But surely the likelihood of hypoxic injury is greater when the flow rate is less, and therefore maximal when the flow rate is zero, i.e. when flow is altogether prevented by double ligation? (Oddly, Wessler scarcely mentioned valves, but as reviewed in the foregoing pages, it was already well established that valves are the sites of venous thrombogenesis.)

As Virchow (1858) remarked, "*the doctrine of stasis rests on manifold misinterpretations*". It is important to re-emphasise his inference that venous thrombi form in *flowing* blood, but not in *static* blood, and that since venous thrombogenesis is a slow process, which may evolve over hours, days or even weeks, the *rate* of blood flow may not be material factor. What matters is that the blood is always 'exchanging', however slowly; moving, rather than stationary for dangerously protracted periods.

Elegant studies on the dynamics of the valve cycle (Lurie *et al.*, 2002, 2003) and the patterns of flow within valve pockets (Karino & Motomiya, 1984; Karino, 1986; Karino & Goldsmith,

1987) helped to resolve the seeming paradox. Essentially, these studies showed that when venous blood flow is *non-pulsatile (streamline)*, as when the patient's 'calf muscle pump' is inactive and there is no intermittent (*vis a tergo*) upward pressure on the soles of the feet, as in walking, a significant part of the blood within 'backwater' valve pockets is not exchanged with the luminal blood. Under such non-pulsatile flow conditions the valve does not execute its usual cycle but remains half-open/half-closed indefinitely.

Near the mouth of the valve pocket, the blood is likely to circulate in a spiral vortex, driven by the laminar flow in the vein lumen. Deep in the pocket is a secondary vortex, rotating in the opposite sense to the primary vortex and more slowly (see Fig. 1). Because the blood in this secondary vortex is never evacuated from the valve pocket while flow in the vein remains non-pulsatile, it becomes increasingly hypoxaemic. Therefore, the endothelia lining the depths of the valve pockets are progressively at risk of hypoxic injury when the venous blood flow is non-pulsatile, *irrespective of the flow rate*. This was demonstrated experimentally by Hamer *et al.* (1981), as discussed below. We concur with Schina *et al.* (1993) that non-pulsatile flow, not slow flow or 'stasis', promotes DVT.

Valve cusp leaflets are avascular (Franklin, 1937; Saphir & Lev, 1952a,b; Sevitt, 1974) - they have no vasa venarum. The outer (medial) endothelial surface (luminalis) is oxygenated by the blood flowing through the vein lumen, irrespective of pulsatility, but the inner, lateral endothelium (parietalis) lining the valve pocket is not (see Fig. 1). Therefore, the parietalis endothelium is at greatest risk of hypoxic injury, and potentially of necrotic cell death, when oxygen-starved during sustained non-pulsatile blood flow.

4.2 The VCH thesis of aetiology: a summary

The initial version of the VCH hypothesis was conceived in 1966 and first outlined in 1977 (Malone, 1977). Its premises were tested critically during the late 1970s and early 1980s. The full version of the validated thesis, with detailed historical and experimental support and scientific and clinical implications, was published some 20 years later (Malone & Agutter, 2006, 2008). The VCH thesis is summarised in Figs. 1-4.

Under normal (pulsatile) blood flow conditions, the venous valve pockets are emptied and refilled regularly and thus do not become hypoxaemic (Fig. 1). However, if there is sustained non-pulsatile ('streamline') venous blood flow, DVT may occur. Such flow leads to suffocating hypoxaemia in the venous valve pockets, resulting in hypoxic injury to the inner (parietalis) endothelium of the cusp leaflets (Fig. 2).

This hypoxic injury activates the pleiotropic elk-1/egr-1 pathway within the endothelial cells, which in turn activates a number of chemoattractant and procoagulant factors. When normal pulsatile blood flow is restored, even transiently, leukocytes and platelets, attracted by these factors, may swarm to the site of dead endothelial cells and initiate protective coagulant action locally (Fig. 3).

Prolongation of non-pulsatile flow for multiple hours may kill the accumulated blood cells in the unemptied valve pocket. These dead cells may then form the core of a nascent thrombus (Fig. 4). If periods of non-pulsatile and pulsatile flow continue to alternate in that abnormal sequential pattern (very protracted stasis + very brief normal flow), the ensuing serial deposition of white cells may contribute the most distinctive morphological characteristic of a venous thrombus, the striking Lines of Zahn.

Subsequent dehiscence of the growing thrombus, with or without the necrotic endothelial layer to which it is attached, might explain why venous thrombi embolise so readily. The VCH thesis also provides an aetiological explanation for post-thrombotic syndrome and, indeed, for chronic venous insufficiency in general (Malone & Agutter, 2009).

4.3 Validation of the VCH thesis

The original VCH hypothesis led to two readily testable predictions, which were the subjects of experimental studies during the 1980s. The results of these studies were unequivocal:

1. deliberately (artificially) sustained non-pulsatile flow in human patients under anaesthesia causes extreme hypoxaemia in the valve pockets, which results in hypoxia extending to anoxia in the blood 'servicing' endothelial cells in the distal pockets;
2. sustained non-pulsatile flow alternating with brief episodes of pulsatile flow in experimental animals, also under anaesthesia, generates thrombi that are morphologically indistinguishable from autochthonous venous thrombi.

The first prediction was examined on a series of patients undergoing surgery for varicose veins (Hamer *et al.*, 1981). In accordance with standard practice, the anaesthetist maintained normal circulating PO_2 levels in these patients. However, the PO_2 in the valve pockets fell consistently, and when the oxygen electrode was brought into contact with the endothelial surface lining at the base of the pockets, there was no response. The PO_2 level in these cells had fallen to a value below the detection limit of the electrode, not only confirming the predicted hypoxaemia in the valve pocket blood during sustained non-pulsatile flow (the circulating blood being still normally oxygenated), but *a fortiori* showing that the valve cusp leaflet is effectively impermeable to oxygen.

The second prediction was tested on dogs that breathed normally after a single dose anaesthetic injection, which by paralysing all muscle-pumping other than respiratory excursions ensured that blood flow in the limbs was non-pulsatile (Hamer & Malone, 1984). When the dogs began to awaken at successive intervals, the legs exhibited 'auto-jactitation' (clonus), each spasm sufficient to pump fresh blood containing living leukocytes and platelets into the recently hypoxaemic valve pockets. X-rays of the upper thigh veins using contrast radiography then revealed the growth of thrombi, which were microscopically/ morphologically indistinguishable from autochthonous venous thrombi.

The significance of these experimental findings was acknowledged by Hume (1985), who stated that the aetiology of DVT was now elucidated. The explanation of venous thrombogenesis in terms of valve cusp hypoxia was empirically demonstrated, no longer a mere hypothesis. (Hume, a surgeon who specialised in DVT, had co-authored a major monograph on the subject with Sevitt and Thomas in 1970.)

There is a third prediction, which without the VCH thesis might seem counterintuitive: it is that thrombi may form in limb veins should *rapid* blood flow remain non-pulsatile for extended periods. This prediction could repay testing on experimental animals; a convincing experiment would be instructive, though it would be technically difficult to conduct.

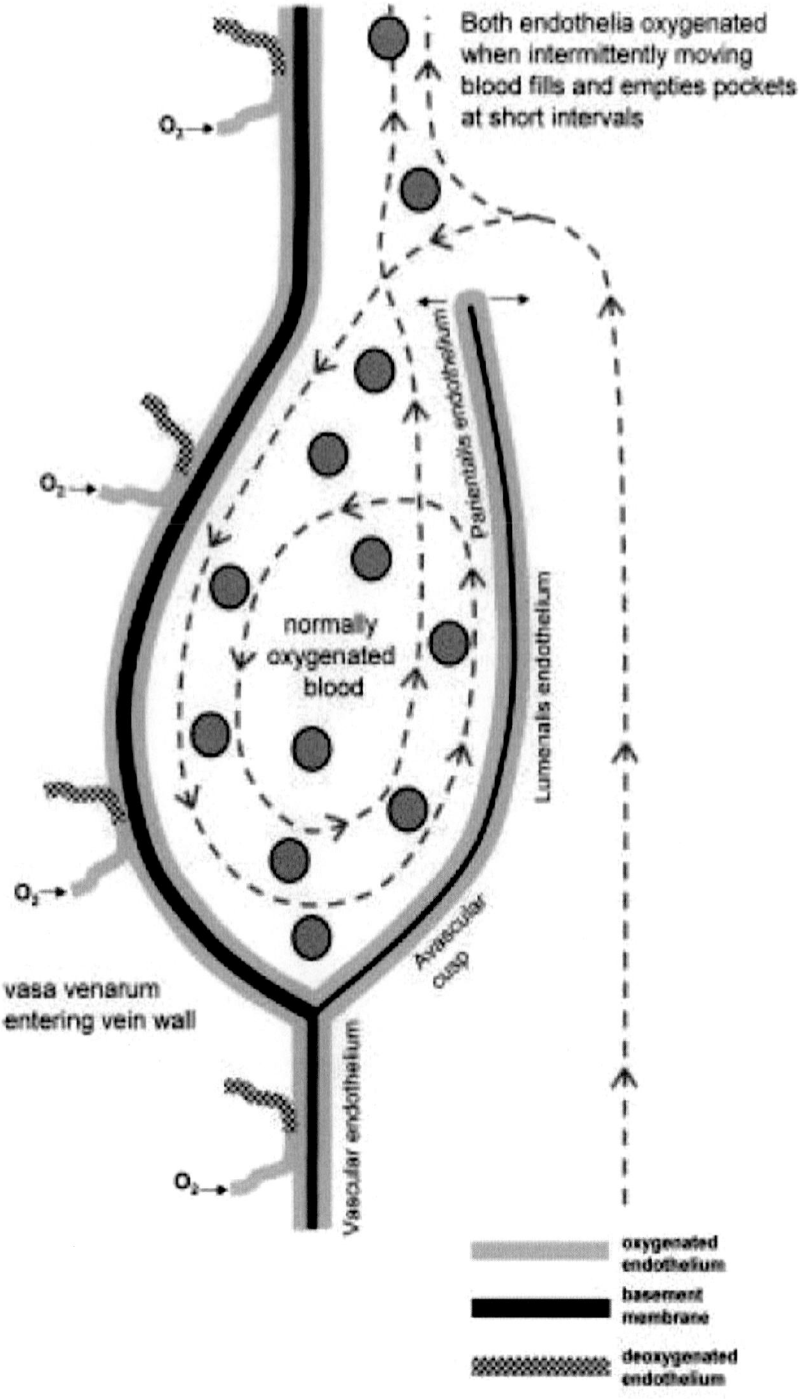

Fig. 1. Blood movements within and around a venous valve pocket during normal (pulsatile flow) conditions. The blood in the pocket exchanges regularly with the luminal blood, so valve pocket hypoxaemia does not develop and the endothelia lining the pocket remain oxygenated.

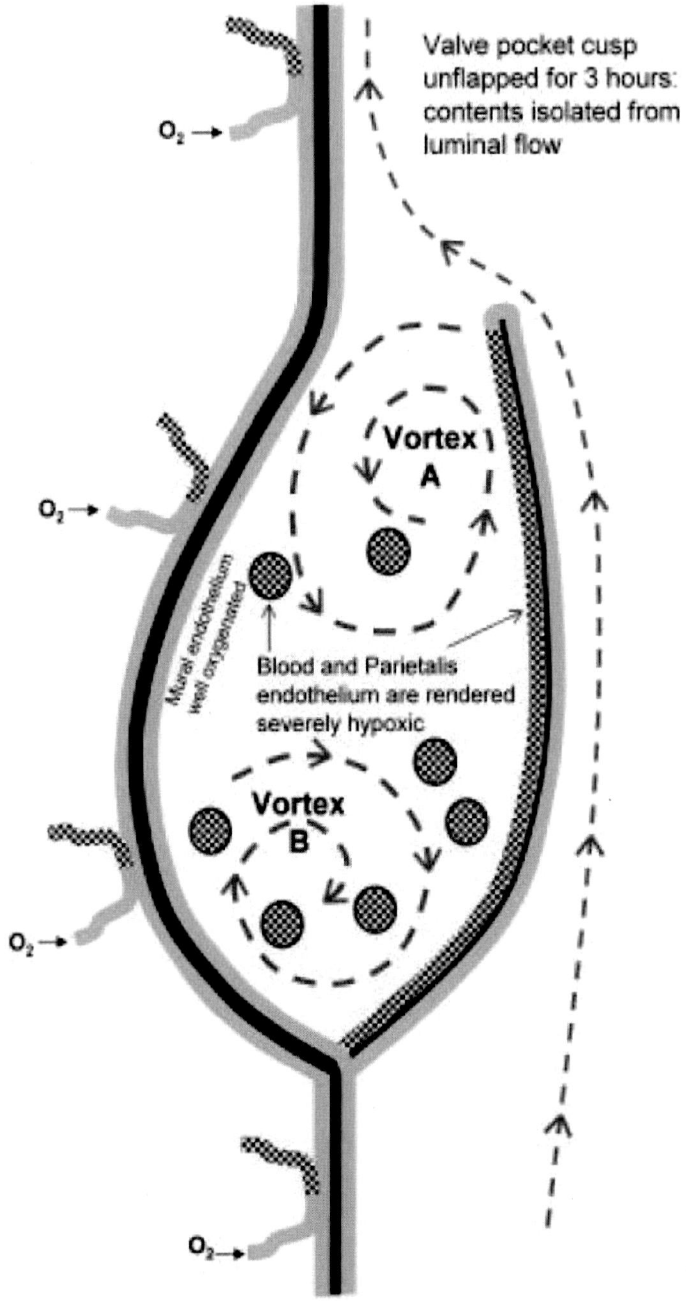

Fig. 2. When blood flow along the vein becomes non-pulsatile, irrespective of speed, the blood in the valve pocket is no longer exchanged with luminal blood, as it is under normal pulsatile flow conditions (Fig. 1). The laminar flow past the mouth of the valve pocket drives a vortex (A) in the upper part of the pocket, and this in turn drives a secondary vortex (B), rotating very slowly in the opposite sense, in the depths of the pocket. Local hypoxaemia leads to severe hypoxia, especially of the parietalis endothelium.

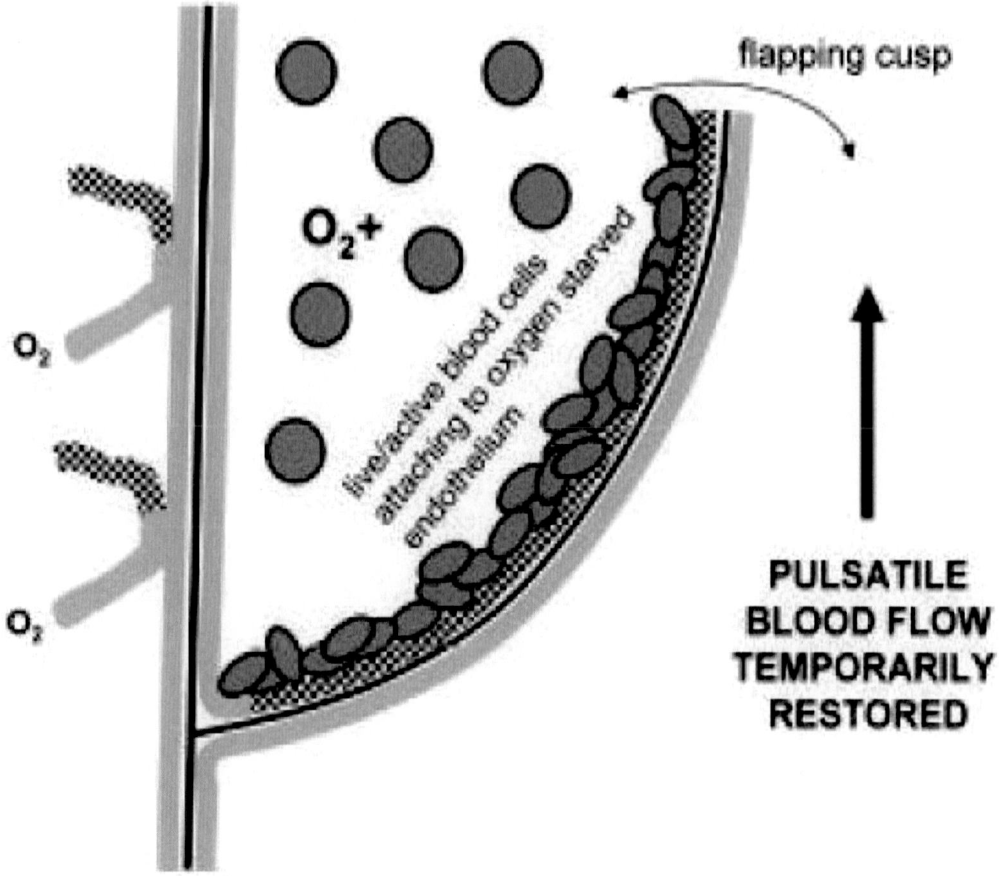

Fig. 3. Each single pulsation by the muscle pump will evacuate 'dead blood' from all affected valve pockets after prolonged periods of hypoxaemia and replace it with fresh blood containing living, active white cells including platelets. In this diagrammatic illustration, these fresh cells are shown in juxtaposition with the parietalis endothelium; our evidence and the historical literature (Aschoff, 1924; Saphir & Lev, 1952a; Sevitt, 1974) indicate that leukocytes swarm on to the severely embarrassed or possibly dead/ necrotic cell layer, forming the white core of the thrombus *Kopfteil*. Because the valve leaflet projects into the centre of the vein, the *Kopfteil* may have seemed to its first observers to be 'in the centre of the afflicted vein'. It may be conjectured that the vein wall endothelial cells deep in the valve pocket also become sufficiently hypoxic for the egr-1 pathway to be activated, notwithstanding any possible oxygenation via the vasa venarum. This is assumed by Bovill & van der Vleet (2011), who propose that coagulation is initiated on the vein wall endothelium, not the valve cusp parietalis, a speculation that will be discussed further in section 5.

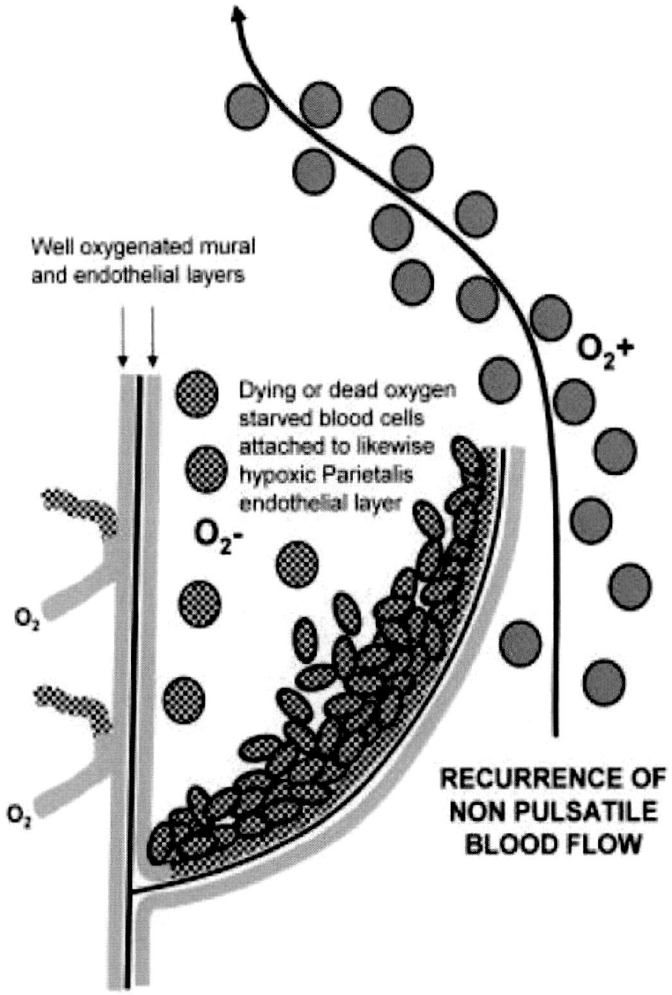

Fig. 4. When sustained non-pulsatile flow resumes after a pulsatile episode, any white cells that have swarmed over the necrotic parietalis endothelium die likewise as a result of valve pocket hypoxaemia. Meanwhile, coagulation can continue. With further episodes of pulsatile flow, the process will be repeated, generating successive layerings of dead cells interspersed with fibrin, accounting for the Lines of Zahn morphology. The necrotic parietalis is fragile and is liable to dehisce (see illustrations in Malone & Agutter, 2008, chapter 10), particularly when the nascent thrombus outgrows the valve pocket and protrudes into the vein lumen, where it is subjected to tension by the flowing blood after the resumption of pulsatility. This may explain the tendency of venous thrombi to embolise.

5. Extending the VCH thesis of aetiology

5.1 Accounting for Virchow's *real* triad

As previously elaborated (Malone & Agutter, 2006, 2008), the VCH explains leukocyte accumulation and the white *Kopfteil*, it accounts for most of the known risk factors such as the effect of ageing (cf. Saphir & Lev, 1952b; Van Langevelde *et al.*, 2010), and it is consistent with the readiness of venous thrombi to embolise. However, though it is consistent with them, some might reserve judgment as to whether it accounts fully and explicitly for (1) the high density of the fibrin around the *Kopfteil* and (2) the Lines of Zahn. These observations need further clarification.

The dense fibrin in nascent thrombi was likewise described by Sevitt (1974). Bovill & van der Vliet (2011) pointed out that it is consistent with tissue factor (TF)-induced coagulation, but they suggested that coagulation is initiated on the vein wall not the parietalis endothelium of the valve pocket. That suggestion would have to be experimentally verified and corroborated before it could be regarded as fact rather than conjecture. Its plausibility depends on the commonly held belief that TF is the primary physiological trigger for coagulation (e.g. Hoffman & Monroe, 2001); also, TF is one of the many targets of activation by egr-1 (Mechtcheriakova *et al.*, 1999) so it is expected that valve pocket hypoxaemia will activate it. Primary involvement of TF in coagulation during venous thrombogenesis could explain why anticoagulants are allegedly more effective for prophylaxis than are platelet inhibitors.

A possible difficulty with this explanation for the high fibrin density is that heparin does not inhibit the initiation of thrombi on hypoxic venous endothelium (Samuels & Webster, 1952), and heparin is known to inhibit TF directly and by activating tissue factor promoting inhibitor (e.g. Lupu *et al.*, 1999; Ettalaie *et al.*, 2011). Alternative explanations should therefore be considered. For instance, the inception and growth of a venous thrombus are slow processes, characterised by the serial margination of successive layers of platelets and leukocytes on the hypoxia-induced lesion of the valve pocket endothelium as blood continues to circulate past the site. This results in a much denser crowding of platelets (as well as leukocytes) than is likely in a haemostatic plug or during the coagulation of shed blood, and densely crowded platelets will generate a dense fibrin mesh.

No matter whether coagulation is TF-induced by the luminal endothelial cells of the valve pocket, as Bovill & van der Vliet speculate, or whether the crowded platelets on and around the injured/ necrotic parietalis endothelium spin out the dense fibrin, logical extension of the VCH thesis provides an explanation for that facet of Virchow's *real* triad. As for the Lines of Zahn, the serial deposition described earlier is the critical factor; but the slow secondary vortex in the depths of the valve pocket (Karino, 1986) will also contribute by weaving the leukocyte/platelet-rich and dense fibrin layers around each other.

Thus, the extended VCH mechanism accounts for all three aspects of Virchow's *real* triad.

5.2 Cross-talk between leukocyte recruitment and coagulation

The molecular changes in endothelial cells subjected to valve pocket hypoxaemia were discussed in chapter 12 of Malone & Agutter (2008) and by Bovill & van der Vliet (2011). The generation of reactive oxygen species (ROS) in the hypoxic endothelium is of particular interest because ROS promote both neutrophil recruitment (Millar *et al.*, 2007) and the activation of TF (Banfi *et al.*, 2009), as well as activating egr-1. This involvement of ROS could support the proposal that a vegan diet has prophylactic value against DVT and VTE (Cundiff *et al.*, 2010), since vegan diets are allegedly rich in antioxidants, though a statistically sound test of this proposal would involve a very large patient cohort. Bovill & van der Vliet note that other hypoxia-related transcription factors such as hypoxia-inducible factor-1 are potential targets for ROS in the affected endothelium, though the relevance of this to venous thrombogenesis is uncertain.

In examining the molecular cross-talk between leukocyte recruitment and coagulation during venous thrombogenesis, it is important to distinguish early events from developments associated with the growth of a 'mature' thrombus. For example, TF-bearing microvesicles derived from either monocytes or vein wall pericytes seem to be prominent during the development of thrombi, but are almost certainly not involved during the initiation of venous thrombosis (Bovill & van der Vliet, 2011). More importantly from the practical, clinical standpoint, anticoagulants stop the growth of a thrombus but they do not prevent its initiation. It is therefore not surprising that the decline in incidence of DVT/VTE and post-thrombotic syndrome in hospital patients has been only marginal, notwithstanding recent advances in anticoagulant treatment (Kahn & Ginsberg, 2004; Heit, 2005).

5.3 Why is DVT not even more common than it is?

The evidence reviewed in section 4 testifies to the correctness of the VCH thesis, but the imaginative reader might raise this question. Sustained non-pulsatile flow in the deep limb veins with short episodes of pulsatile flow are quite common in the daily lives of some humans, and is certainly common among carnivores, which sleep and remain immobile for many hours per day. In this context, the proposal of Brooks *et al.* (2009) that the valve pocket endothelia are more resistant than the luminal endothelium to the induction of coagulation could be of interest.

These authors proposed, on the basis of preliminary evidence, that the levels of von Willebrand factor (vWF), thrombomodulin (TM) and endothelial protein C receptor (EPCR) change with depth in the valve pocket, so that the endothelial cells express less of the procoagulant (vWF) and more of the anticoagulant (TM and EPCR) factors. Trotman *et al.* (2011) pursued this hypothesis and found that the level of vWF did indeed decrease with depth in the pocket, but so did the level of EPCR; the TM level showed no significant change. There was extensive inter-individual variation in all three of these proteins, so the patterns were not entirely clear, but the hypothesis advanced by these authors could in principle help to explain 'why DVT is not even more common than it is'. In principle, The Brooks *et al.* proposal could be tested critically by a study on a large experimental animal group. The incidence of thrombogenesis under conditions similar to those used by Hamer & Malone (1984) could be correlated with the expression of vWF (and perhaps TM and EPCR), as assessed e.g. by immunostaining in the valve pocket endothelia after the end of the experiment. However, the most important factor in thrombogenesis is without doubt the duration of the valve pocket hypoxaemia.

6. Implications of the VCH mechanism for prophylaxis

6.1 The balance between anticoagulant and mechanical prophylaxis should be reconsidered

Anticoagulants do not prevent the initiation of DVT (section 5.2), in particular the recruitment and margination of leukocytes and platelets to the injured parietalis endothelium, but they prevent the growth of already-formed venous thrombi to clinically significant size. Whether they inhibit the putative local effects of TF (see above) is debatable.

From the point of view of patient care, this is not a crucial issue; what is important is to prevent the potential morbidity and mortality associated with DVT, specifically VTE and post-thrombotic syndrome. Therefore, preventing thrombus growth is 'useful'. Nevertheless, it seems inherently more satisfactory to prevent the initiation of thrombosis rather than just thrombus growth. That entails a reconsideration of mechanical rather than anticoagulant prophylaxis.

However, current approaches to mechanical prophylaxis are unlikely to achieve the objective of preventing the initiation of thrombogenesis. The NICE website sums up the conventional explanation for the effects of intermittent pneumatic compression, though with a curious use of the word 'theory': "*The theory behind mechanical approaches to thromboprophylaxis is that they increase mean blood flow velocity in leg veins, reducing venous stasis*" (National Institute for Clinical Excellence, 2011). It would be valid to presume that an 'adequate' mean venous blood flow velocity maintains our existence and lives, since an 'inadequate' flow velocity would ultimately be incompatible with life; nevertheless, the 'theory' invoked above in support of intermittent pneumatic compression is not consistent with our experimental proof that *pulsatile* flow maintenance is the true thromboprophylactic. The assumption that venous flow velocity has any significance in thrombogenesis is unproven, and according to the VCH thesis it is likely to be false.

This widespread misunderstanding about the significance of venous return blood flow velocity may explain why mechanical prophylaxis has remained adjunctive to anticoagulant treatment. Thus, Khoury *et al.* (2011) describe mechanical prophylaxis as 'inappropriate' or 'inadequate' unless anticoagulation is contraindicated (because of a serious bleeding risk), and authoritative sources such as Demtali *et al.* (2007), Geerts *et al.* (2008) and Sliwka & Fang (2010) strongly support the use of anticoagulant "*and to a lesser degree mechanical*" forms of prophylaxis (the quoted phrase is from Sliwka & Fang, 2010). Similarly, we recall that "*Chemoprophylaxis is recommended for medical patients at moderate to high risk of venous thromboembolism (VTE) and is now a requirement of the Joint Commission on Accreditation of Healthcare Organizations*" (Rothberg *et al.*, 2010). Moreover, a very large international survey by Kakkar *et al.* (2010) revealed that "*Anticoagulant therapy was much more frequently used than mechanical devices such as compression stockings or intermittent pneumatic compression, even in patients at increased risk of bleeding*".

However, the truth - revealed explicitly by modern medical/surgical practice - is that anticoagulants and mechanical prophylaxis work hand in hand. Physicians might be more inclined to emphasise pharmacological approaches and surgeons to emphasise mechanical ones, but the difference is not absolute and the methods need not be considered mutually exclusive. Since prompt ambulation of post-operative surgical patients has also become routine in recent decades (Cundiff *et al.*, 2010), this form of mechanical prophylaxis, which ensures pulsatile return blood flow in the legs, has long been valued in reducing the incidence of post-surgical DVT/VTE alongside anticoagulants; yet it might not have been recognised universally as a form of 'mechanical prophylaxis'.

The VCH thesis does not lead to an argument against anticoagulant prophylaxis. However, long-term anticoagulant use is associated with fatal or disabling bleeding (Cundiff *et al.*, 2010; Cundiff, 2011) and Cochrane reviews make clear that the evidence supporting anticoagulant prophylaxis should be monitored constantly (Cundiff, 2011), and that such prophylaxis against VTE may hypothetically be contraindicated. In a sense, giving a patient anticoagulants 'in case' he/she develops DVT might be seen as akin to dosing such patient with chemotherapeutic drugs 'in case' he/she develops a cancer.

That is an extreme view. Nevertheless, the balance between the anticoagulant and mechanical approaches to prophylaxis needs to be re-evaluated in the light of the VCH thesis, since they seem likely in time to perfect a more impartial 'cross-party' view of the aetiology of DVT and of patient management.

6.2 Mechanical prophylaxis: a rational approach

The simple objective of mechanical prophylaxis is to ensure that blood in the valve pockets is exchanged at regular intervals (Malone & Agutter, 2008). Modern surgical prophylaxis could readily be improved if the VCH principle were added to the classical objective: 'regular' (i.e. regular intermittent) pulsation need not necessarily mean *'as frequent as is current practice'*. In chapter 9 of our monograph we calculated that valve pocket hypoxaemia does not become dangerous (i.e. potentially injurious) until non-pulsatile flow has persisted for 1.5-3 hours, an estimate consistent with the empirical data (Hamer *et al.*, 1981). Less frequent, i.e. *relatively infrequent*, artificial pulses (perhaps once per hour, though that would need experiential confirmation) would preclude thrombogenesis, and would be more comfortable for patients than what must seem incessant limb compression at short intervals, day and night.

For patients confined to prolonged bed-rest, insensible, automatic alternate end-to-end Trendelenberg/ anti-Trendelenberg tilting of the bed, through a 5-10 degree angle, every hour or so, should be prophylactic by emptying the valve pockets in the upper and lower parts of the body by gravity, allowing them to refill passively with fresh venous blood at relatively short intervals (as above) and preventing unsuspected but potentially fatal hypoxaemia in unmoved pockets.

6.3 Testing the proposals for rational mechanical prophylaxis

Preferably, these proposals would require further animal testing before clinical deployment. Perhaps the original experimental design created and used by Hamer & Malone (1984) would suffice as a basis.

Three matched groups of anaesthetised animals would be required initially, each to be subjected to prolonged non-pulsatile blood flow in the leg veins, with brief alternating pulsatile episodes: (a) controls, untreated; (b) given standard anticoagulant prophylaxis; (c) given mechanical prophylaxis by one or other of the methods proposed in section 6.2. At the end of the experiment, valves from deep limb veins would be examined microscopically. The VCH prediction would be that group (a) will show the formation of quasi-autochthonous thrombi; group (b) might show incipient thrombi on the parietalis endothelia; and group (c) will show normal endothelia with no incipient thrombi.

Positive results might suggest that a randomised controlled clinical trial of one or both of the approaches outlined in section 6.2 should be undertaken. At the same time, this experimental set-up could provide a means for testing the efficacy of anticoagulants in absolute terms; for the past 50 years, anticoagulant prophylaxis has been evaluated only by statistical evidence, without the use of such a 'measuring rod'.

6.4 Application of rational mechanical prophylactic measures

In the absence of contrary evidence, there is a *prima facie* case for using the measures described in section 6.2 throughout the period of bed rest for all acute medical patients and for surgical patients with limited mobility. That would be in line with the recommendations of NICE in the UK, of similar bodies in other European countries, and of the Joint Commission on Accreditation of Healthcare Organizations in the USA (see earlier discussion), except that anticoagulants would be given a less central role in prophylaxis. (There would be little or no need for any such measures in ambulant patients.)

One area that might need more or less radical reconsideration is surgery involving general anaesthesia. However, we emphasise that our comments here are conjectural and would require detailed evaluation before they were considered for practical application. Also, they relate to a potential risk associated only with very prolonged anaesthesia, involving sustained muscle relaxation, not to surgical operations in general.

It is self-evident that relaxant anaesthesia is inherently thrombogenic. For short operations, this is unlikely to matter greatly; but for longer operations (say over 100 minutes) during which the patient is totally motionless, there is a major risk that undetectable prothrombogenic nidi will form in valve pockets. The muscular paralysis induced during anaesthesia will therefore cause thrombosis in every case unless the duration of the resultant streamline (non-pulsatile) blood flow in all veins of the body is constantly kept in mind. If the unconscious patient's veins are not squeezed, e.g. by mechanical movement of limbs, then valve pocket hypoxaemia cannot be avoided. In reality, of course, the risk depends on how quickly the patient recovers from the effects of the muscle relaxant so that the skeletal muscles of the limbs start to contract again. It would seem ideal for the state of total muscle paralysis to last only ½ to ¾ of an hour, after which the anaesthetist would have to administer another dose of curare, but that is speculation; confirmation from practice and experience would be essential before such proposals were applied.

All anaesthetists are acutely aware of the respiratory support (sustained oxygen supply) needed for safe anaesthesia, but they are far less likely to be concerned about the restoration of pulsatile blood flow in the patient's legs/ abdomen. Appropriate practice must relate to the acceptability of temporary recovery of patient motion to the surgeon, and of course the delicacy of the operation and the disturbance likely from any change in anaesthetic practice.

Besides monitoring relaxant anaesthesia, the practice of end-to-end Trendelenburg/anti-Trendenburg tilting discussed in section 6.2 could be re-employed. However, the number of degrees elevation and reduction would be only 2 x 5% to and fro in 'horizontal patient' operations. Operations performed e.g. in sitting positions would require different manoeuvres appropriate to the particular patient posture. The objective in all cases would be to limit drugged-immobility to a specific duration that must be established by experience (after an initial informed guess based on e.g. the evidence from Hamer *et al.*, 1981).

7. Conclusions

The currently prevailing beliefs about the aetiology of DVT arose from the assumption, fostered by the ascent of haematology after the Second World War, that venous thrombogenesis is primarily (or exclusively) a matter of *in situ* blood coagulation. This view became associated with a misreading of Virchow's work that gave rise to 'Virchow's triad';

an ironic association, since a key aspect of Virchow's work on venous thrombi was his three-part distinction between thrombus and clot and his demonstration that a DVT is formed when leukocytes as well as platelets swarm to the site of injury, the venous valve cusp. As a result, mainstream research in the DVT field since 1962 has taken on an increasingly haematological character, which has entailed a tacit dismissal of the important discoveries made prior to the mid-20th century, not least those of Virchow. The valve cusp hypoxia (VCH) thesis is founded on the recognition of these discoveries and on our knowledge of vascular physiology, particularly the dynamics of blood flow in venous valve pockets. It was advanced as a hypothesis in 1977 and was corroborated and validated by critical experiments during the 1980s.

In clinical terms, the VCH thesis adds nothing to accepted standards of treatment for actual, manifest thromboembolism other than to augment the rational basis for mechanical prophylaxis and to suggest reconsideration of prolonged muscle relaxant use during surgery, a potential 'silent killer'. Mechanical prophylaxis should be based not on altering the venous blood flow velocity, which is almost certainly irrelevant to thrombogenesis, but to ensuring that flow is always pulsatile. The pulses need not be frequent: once per hour will suffice to ensure that valve pocket hypoxaemia does not become seriously injurious to the endothelia, and should therefore preclude the formation of thrombi, though optimal timing can only be established on the basis of experience. The key point is to ensure that the valve pockets are emptied and refilled regularly with fresh venous blood. On the other hand, the VCH thesis indicates that anticoagulants do not prevent the initiation of deep venous thrombosis, though they restrict or retard the growth of thrombi that have already formed.

The approaches to mechanical prophylaxis inferred from VCH are testable on experimental animals. Such tests should certainly be conducted before a randomised controlled clinical trial is initiated. We encourage colleagues throughout the world to undertake these experiments - and, subject to the results, clinical trials - since only by consistent findings from different laboratories and clinical establishments can a consensus be obtained that would make rational mechanical prophylaxis the standard of care for patients at risk for DVT/ VTE.

8. References

Agutter, P.S. & Malone, P.C. (2011). Deep Venous Thrombosis: Hunter, Cruveilhier, Virchow, and present-day understanding and clinical practice. *International Journal of the History and Philosophy of Medicine* Vol. 1, pp. 7-14

Anderson, J.A. & Weitz, J.I. (2010). Hypercoagulable states. *Clinics in Chest Medicine* Vol. 31, No. 4 (December), pp. 659-673, ISSN 0272-5231

Anning, S.T. (1957). The historical aspects of venous thrombosis. *Medical History* Vol. 1, No. 1 (January), pp. 28-37, ISSN 0025-7273

Arya, R. (2011) The National VTE prevention programme, In: Venous Embolism Prevention , accessed 15 July 2011, Available from: http://kingsthrombosiscentre.org.uk/kings/multimedia/nationalvteprevention/arya/index.htm

Aschoff, L. (1924). *Lectures in General Pathology*, Hoeber, New York

Asherton, R.A. & Hughes, G.R. (1989). Recurrent deep vein thrombosis and Addison's disease in 'primary' antiphospholipid syndrome. *The Journal of Rheumatology*, Vol. 16, No. 3 (March), pp. 378-380, ISSN 0315-162X

Bagot, C.N. & Arya, R. (2008). Virchow and his triad: a question of attribution. *British Journal of Haematology,* Vol. 143, No. 2 (October), pp. 180-190, ISSN 0007-1048

Banfi, C., Brioschi, M., Barbieri, S.S., Eligini, S., Barcella, S., Tremoli, E., Colli, S. & Mussoni, L. (2009). Mitochondrial reactive oxygen species: a common pathway for PAR1- and PAR2-mediated TF induction in human endothelial cells. *Journal of Thrombosis and Haemostasis,* Vol. 7, No. 1 (January), pp. 206–216, ISSN 1538-7933

Baumgarten, P. (1876). Űber die Sog. Organisation des Thrombus. *Zentralblatt für den medizinische Wissenschaft,* Vol. 14, pp. 593-597

Berna, N.; Arnould, T.; Remacle, J. & Michiels, C. (2001). Hypoxia-induced increase in calcium concentration in endothelial cells: role of the Na^+-glucose cotransporter. *Journal of Cellular Biochemistry,* Vol. 84, No. 1, pp. 115-131, ISSN 0730-2312

Biggs, R. & MacFarlane, R.G. (1962). *Human Blood Coagulation and its Disorders,* 3rd edition, Blackwell, Oxford

Bovill, E.G. & van der Vliet, A. (2011). Venous valvular stasis-associated hypoxia and thrombosis: what is the link? *Annual Review of Physiology,* Vol. 73, pp. 527-545, ISSN 0066-4278

Brinkhous, K.M. (1969). The problem in perspective, In: *Thrombosis,* Sherry, S. (ed.), pp. 37-48, National Academy of Sciences, Washington

Brooks, E.G.; Trotman, W.; Wadsworth, M.P.; Taatjes, D.J.; Evans, M.F.; Ittleman, F.P.; Callas, P.W.; Esmon, C.T. & Bovill, E.G. (2009). Valves of the deep venous system: an overlooked risk factor. *Blood,* Vol. 114, No. 6 (August), pp. 1276-1279, ISSN 0006-4971

Brotman, D.J.; Deitcher, S.R.; Lip, G.Y. & Matzdorff, A.C. (2004). Virchow's triad revisited. *Southern Medical Journal,* Vol. 97, No. 2 (February), pp. 213-214

Bulger, C.M.; Jacobs, C. & Patel, N.H. (2004). Epidemiology of acute deep vein thrombosis. *Techniques in Vascular and Interventional Radiology,* Vol. 7, No. 2, (June), pp. 50-54, ISSN 1089-2516

Comerota, A.J.; Stewart, G.J. & White, J.V. (1985). Combined dihydroergotamine and heparin prophylaxis of postoperative deep vein thrombosis: proposed mechanism of action. *American Journal of Surgery,* Vol. 150, No. 4A (October), pp. 39-44, ISSN 0002-9610

Cundiff, D.K.; Agutter, P.S.; Malone, P.C. & Pezzullo, J. (2010). Diet as prophylaxis and treatment for venous thromboembolism? *Theoretical Biology and Medical Modelling,* Vol. 7 (August), paper 31, ISSN 1742-4682

Cundiff, D.K. (2011). *Whistleblower Doctor: The Politics and Economics of Pain and Dying.* Los Angeles, CA, ISBN 0-9761571-3-6, Private publication

Dentali, F.; Douketis, J.D.; Gianni, M.; Lim, W. & Crowther, M.A. (2007). Meta-analysis: Anticoagulant prophylaxis to prevent symptomatic venous thromboembolism in hospitalized medical patients. *Annals of Internal Medicine, Vol.* 146, No. 4 (), pp. 278–288, ISSN 0003-4819

Dickson, B.C. (2004). Venous thrombosis: on the history of Virchow's triad. *University of Toronto Medical Journal,* Vol. 81, pp. 166-171, ISSN 0042-0239

Drinker, C.K. (1938). *Carbon Monoxide Asphyxia.* Oxford University Press, New York (see especially pp. 124 ff)

Eagle, H. (1938). Recent advances in the blood coagulation problem. *Medicine,* Vol. 16, pp. 95-138

Egeberg, O. (1965). Inherited antithrombin III deficiency causing thrombophilia. *Thrombosis et Diathesis Haemorrhagica,* Vol. 13 (June), pp. 516-530, ISSN 0340-5338

Esmon, C.T. (2009). Basic mechanisms and pathogenesis of venous thrombosis. *Blood Review*, Vol. 23, No. 5 (September), pp. 225-229, ISSN 0268-960X

Ettelaie, C.; Fountain, D.; Collier, M-E.W.; Beeby, E.; Xiao, Y.P. & Maraveyas, A. (2011). Low molecular weight heparin suppresses tissue factor-mediated cancer cell invasion and migration in vitro. *Experimental and Therapeutic Medicine,* Vol. 2, No. 1 (January), pp. 363-367, ISSN 1792-0981

Franklin, K.J. (1937). *A Monograph on Veins*. Charles Thomas, Springfield, Illinois, chapter 5

Geerts, W.H.; Pineo, G.F.; Heit, J.A.; Bergqvist, D.; Lassen, M.R.; Colwell, C.W. & Ray, J.G. (2004). Prevention of venous thromboembolism: the seventh ACCP Conference on antithrombotic and thrombolytic therapy. *Chest,* Vol. 126, Supplement 3 (September), pp. 338S-400S, ISSN 0012-3692

Geerts, W.H.; Bergqvist, D.; Pineo, G.F.; Heit, J.A.; Samama, C.M.; Lassen, M.R. & Colwell, C.W. American College of Chest Physicians. (2008). Prevention of venous thromboembolism: American college of chest physicians evidence-based clinical practice guidelines (8th edition). Chest, Vol. 133, No. 6 Suppl (June), pp. 381S–453S, ISSN 0012-3692

Gibbs, N.M. (1957). Venous thrombosis in the lower limbs with particular reference to bed rest. *The British Journal of Surgery,* Vol. 45, No. 191 (November), pp. 209-236, ISSN 0007-1323

Hamby, R.I. (2005). Deep Vein Thrombosis, In *Heart Center Online website,* accessed 2nd November 2007, Available from: www.heartcenteronline.com

Hamer, J.D.; Malone, P.C. & Silver, I.A. (1981). The PO_2 in venous valve pockets: its possible bearing on thrombogenesis. *The British Journal of Surgery,* Vol. 68, No. 3 (March), pp. 166-170, ISSN 0007-1323

Hamer, J.D. & Malone, P.C. (1984). Experimental deep venous thrombogenesis by a non-invasive method. *Annals of the Royal College of Surgeons of England,* Vol. 66, No. 6 (November), pp. 416–419, ISSN 0035-8843

Harvey, W. (1628). *Exercitatio anatomica de motu cordis et sanguinis in animalibus,* Frankfort. Trans. Willis, R. (1910). *On the Motion of the Heart and Blood in Animals,* Harvard Classics vol. 38, Collier and Son, New York

Hassouna, H.I. (2009). Thrombophilia and hypercoagulability. *Medical Principles and Practice (Kuwait),* Vol. 18, No. 6 (December), pp. 429-440, ISSN 1011-7571

Heit, J.A. (2005). Venous thromboembolism: disease burden, outcomes and risk factors. *Journal of Thrombosis and Haemostasis,* Vol. 3, No. 8 (August), pp. 1611–1617, ISSN 1538-7933

Hewson, W. (1771). *An Experimental Enquiry into the Properties of Blood.* London, T. Cadell, p. 20

Hoffman, M. & Monroe, D.M. 3rd. (2001). A cell-based model of hemostasis. *Thrombosis and Haemostasis,* Vol. 85, No. 6 (June), pp. 958–965, ISSN 0340-6245

Hume, M. (1985). Re. Experimental deep venous thrombogenesis by a non-invasive method. *Annals of the Royal College of Surgeons of England,* Vol. 67, No. 4 (July), p. 268, ISSN 0035-8843

Hunter, J. (1793). Observations on the inflammation of the internal coats of veins. *Transactions of the Society for the Improvement of Medical and Chirurgical Knowledge,* Vol. 1, pp. 18-41

Jackson R.M.; Ann, H.S. & Oparil, S. (1988). Hypoxia-induced oxygen tolerance: maintenance of endothelial metabolic function. *Experimental Lung Research*, Vol. 14, Supplement, pp. 887-896, ISSN 0190-2148

Kahn, S.R. & Ginsberg, J.S. (2004). Relationship between deep venous thrombosis and the postthrombotic syndrome. *Archives of Internal Medicine,* Vol. 164, No. 1 (January), pp. 17–26, ISSN 0003-9926

Kakkar, A.K.; Cohen, A.T.; Tapson, V.F.; Bergmann, J.F.; Goldhaber, S.Z.; Deslandes, B.; Huang, W. & Anderson, F.A. Jr. ENDORSE Investigators. (2010). Venous thromboembolism risk and prophylaxis in the acute care hospital setting (ENDORSE Survey): findings in surgical patients. *Annals of Surgery* Vol. 251, No. 2 (February), pp. 330-338, ISSN 0003-4932

Karimova, A. & Pinsky, D.J. (2001). The endothelial response to oxygen deprivation: biology and clinical implications. *Intensive Care Medicine,* Vol. 27, No. 1 (January), pp. 19-31, ISSN 0342-4642

Karino, T. (1986). Microscopic structure of disturbed flows in the arterial and venous systems, and its implication in the localization of vascular diseases. *International Angiology,* Vol. 5, No. 4 (October-December), pp. 297-313, ISSN 0392-9590

Karino, T. & Goldsmith, H.L. (1987). Rheological factors in thrombosis and haemostasis, In *Haemostasis and Thrombosis,* Bloom, A.L. & Thomas, D.P. (eds.), chapter 42, Churchill Livingstone, ISBN 0-443-0-3190-8, Edinburgh

Karino, T. & Motomiya, M. (1984). Flow through a venous valve and its implications for thrombus formation. *Thrombosis Research,* Vol. 36, No. 3 (November), pp. 245-257, ISSN 0049-3848

Khoury, H.; Welner, S.; Kubin, M.;, Folkerts, K. & Haas, S. (2011). Disease burden and unmet needs for prevention of venous thromboembolism in medically ill patients in Europe show underutilization of preventive therapies. *Thrombosis and Haemostasis,* Vol. 106, No. 4 (August), ISSN 0340-6245

Kyrle, P.A. & Eichinger, S. (2009). Is Virchow's triad complete? *Blood,* Vol. 114, No. 6 (August), pp. 1138-1139, ISSN 0006-4971

Lane, D.A.; Mannucci, P.M.; Bauer, K.A.; Bertina, R.M.; Bochkov, N.P.; Boulyjenkov, V.; Changy, M.; Dahlback, B.; Binter, E.K.; Miletich, J.P.; Rosendaal, F.R. & Selgsohn, U. (1996). Inherited thrombophilia. *Thrombosis and Haemostasis,* Vol. 76, No. 5 (November), pp. 651-662; and No. 6 (December), pp. 824-834, ISSN 0340-6245

Lippi, G. & Franchini, M. (2008). Pathogenesis of venous thromboembolism: when the cup runneth over. *Seminars in Thrombosis and Hemostasis,* Vol. 34, No. 8 (November), pp. 747-761, ISSN 0094-6176

Lister, J.L. (1863). Croonian Lecture: On the coagulation of the blood. *Proceedings of the Royal Society,* Vol. 13, pp. 355-364

López, J.A. & Chen, J. (2009). Pathophysiology of venous thrombosis. *Thrombosis Research,* Vol. 123, Supplement 4, pp. S30-34, ISSN 0049-3848

Lupu, C.; Poulsen, E.; Roquefeuil, S.; Westmuckett, A.D.; Kakkar, V.V. & Lupu, F. (1999). Cellular effects of heparin on the production and release of tissue factor pathway inhibitor in human endothelial cells in culture. *Arteriosclerosis, Thrombosis, and Vascular Biology,* Vol. 19, No. 9 (September), pp. 2251-2262, ISSN 1079-5642

Lurie, F.; Kistner, R.L & Eklof, B. (2002). The mechanism of venous valve closure in normal physiologic conditions. *Journal of Vascular Surgery,* Vol. 35, No. 4 (April), pp. 713-717, ISSN 0741-5214

Lurie, F.; Kistner, R.L.; Eklof, B. & Kessler, D. (2003). Mechanism of venous valve closure and the role of the valve in circulation: a new concept. *Journal of Vascular Surgery,* Vol. 38, No. 5 (November), pp. 955-961, ISSN 0741-5214

Malone, P.C. (1977). Hypothesis concerning the aetiology of venous thrombosis. *Medical Hypotheses,* Vol. 3, No. 5 (September-October), pp. 189–201, ISSN 0306-9877

Malone, P.C. & Agutter, P.S. (2006). The aetiology of deep venous thrombosis. *Quarterly Journal of Medicine,* Vol. 99, No. 9 (September), pp. 581-593, ISSN 1460-2725

Malone, P.C. & Agutter, P.S. (2008). *The Aetiology of Deep Venous Thrombosis.* Springer, ISBN 978-1-4020-6649-8, Dordrecht

Malone, P.C. & Agutter, P.S. (2009). To what extent might deep venous thrombosis and chronic venous insufficiency share a common etiology? *International Angiology* Vol. 28, No. 4 (August), ISSN 0392-9590

Malone, P.C. & Morris, C.J. (1978). The sequestration and margination of platelets and leucocytes in veins during conditions of hypokinetic and anaemic hypoxia: potential significance in clinical postoperative venous thrombosis. *Journal of Pathology,* Vol. 125, No. 3 (July), pp. 119-129, ISSN 0022-3417

Malpother, E.D. (1880). Phlebitis of the lower extremities: a secondary complication of injuries to the head. *British Medical Journal,* Vol. 1, p. 483, ISSN 0959-8138

Mammen, E.F. (1992). Pathogenesis of venous thrombosis. *Chest,* Vol. 102, Supplement 6 (December), pp. 640S-644S, ISSN 0012-3692

Mazza, J.J. (2004). Hypercoagulability and venous thromboembolism: a review. *Wisconsin Medical Journal,* Vol. 103, No. 2 (February), pp. 41-49, ISSN 0043-6542

McLachlin, J. & Paterson, J.C. (1951). Some basic observations on venous thrombosis and pulmonary embolism. *Surgery, Gynecology and Obstetrics,* Vol. 93, No. 1 (July), pp. 1-8, ISSN 0039-6087

Mechtcheriakova, D.; Wlachos, A.; Holzmuller, H.; Binder, B.R. & Hofer, E. (1999). Vascular endothelial cell growth factor-induced tissue factor expression in endothelial cells is mediated by EGR-1. *Blood,* Vol. 93, No. 11 (June), pp. 3811–3823, ISSN 0006-4971

Meetoo, D. (2010). In too deep: understanding, detecting and managing DVT. *British Journal of Nursing,* Vol. 19, No. 16 (September), pp. 1021-1027, ISSN 0966-0461

Millar, T.M.; Phan, V. & Tibbles, L.A. (2007). ROS generation in endothelial hypoxia and reoxygenation stimulates MAP kinase signaling and kinase-dependent neutrophil recruitment. *Free Radical Biology and Medicine,* Vol. 42, No. 8 (April), pp. 1165–1177, ISSN 0891-5849

National Institute for Clinical Excellence (2011). Mechanical prophylaxis, In: *Venous Embolism Prevention,* accessed 11 July 2011, Available from: http://kingsthrombosiscentre.org.uk/kings/multimedia/kingsOtherMaterials/mechanicalThromboprophylaxis/index.htm

Ochsner, A.; DeBakey, M.E. & DeCamp, P.T. (1951). Venous thrombosis. Analysis of 580 cases. *Surgery,* Vol. 29, No. 1 (January), pp. 24-43, ISSN 0039-6060

O'Neill, J.F. (1947). The effect on venous endothelium of alterations in blood flow through vessels in vein walls and the possible relation to thrombosis. *Annals of Surgery,* Vol. 126, No. 3 (September), pp. 270-288, ISSN 0003-4932

Owen, C. (2001). *A History of Blood Coagulation*. Mayo Foundation for Medical Education and Research, ISBN 978-1-8930-0590-7, Rochester

Peterson, C. (1986). Venous thrombosis: an overview. *Pharmacotherapy,* Vol. 6, No. 4 part 2 (July-August), pp. 12S-17S, ISSN 0277-0008

Phillips, M.N.; Jones, G.T.; van Rij, A.M. & Zhang, M. (2004). Micro-venous valves in the superficial veins of the human lower limb. *Clinical Anatomy,* Vol. 17, No. 1 (January), pp. 55-60, ISSN 0897-3806

Pinsky, D.J.; Yan, S.-F.; Lawson, C.; Naka, Y.; Chen, J.-X.; Connolly, E.S. Jr. & Stern, D.M. (1995). Hypoxia and modification of the endothelium: implications for regulation of vascular homeostatic properties. *Seminars in Cell Biology,* Vol. 6, No. 5 (October), pp. 283-294, ISSN 1043-4682

Pulvertaft, R.J.V. (1947). Post-operative pulmonary embolism. *Annals of the Royal College of Surgeons of England,* Vol. 1, No. 4 (October), pp. 181-190, ISSN 0035-8843

Robb-Smith, A.H.T. (1955). The Rubicon: changing views on the relationship of thrombosis and blood coagulation. *British Medical Bulletin* Vol. 11, No. 1, pp. 70-77, ISSN 0007-1420

Rosendaal, F.R. (1999). Venous thrombosis: a multicausal disease. *Lancet,* Vol. 353, No. 9159 (April), pp. 1167–1173, ISSN 0140-6736

Rosendaal, F.R. (2005). Venous thrombosis: the role of genes, environment, and behavior. *American Society of Hematology, Education Program*, pp. 1-12, ISSN 1520-4391

Rothberg, M.B.; Lahti, M.; Lekow, P.S. & Lindenauer, P.K. (2010). Venous thromboembolism prophylaxis among medical patients at US hospitals. *Journal of General Internal Medicine,* Vol 25, No. 6 (June), pp. 489-494, ISSN 0884-8734

Samuels, P.B. & Webster, D.R. (1952). The role of venous endothelium in the inception of thrombosis. *Annals of Surgery,* Vol. 136, No. 3 (September), pp. 422-438, ISSN 0003-4932

Sandison, J.C. (1931). Observations on the circulating blood cells, adventitial (Rouget) and muscle cells, endothelium, and macrophages in the transparent chamber of the rabbit's ear. *Anatomical Record,* Vol. 50, pp. 355-379, ISSN 0003-276X

Saphir, O. & Lev, M. (1952a). Venous valvulitis. *Archives of Pathology,* Vol. 53, No. 5 (May), pp. 456-469, ISSN 0363-0153

Saphir, O. & Lev, M. (1952b). The venous valve in the aged. *American Heart Journal,* Vol. 44, No. 6 (December), pp. 843-850, ISSN 0002-8703

Schina, M.J. Jr.; Neumyer, M.M.; Healy, D.A.; Atnip, R.G. & Thiele, B.L. (1993). Influence of age on venous physiologic parameters. *Journal of Vascular Surgery,* Vol. 18, No. 5 (November), pp. 749-752, ISSN 0741-5214

Sevitt, S. (1974). Organization of valve pocket thrombi and the anomalies of double thrombi and valve cusp involvement. *The British Journal of Surgery,* Vol. 61, No. 8 (August), pp. 641-649, ISSN 0007-1323

Sliwka, D. & Fang, M.C. (2010). Venous thromboembolism prophylaxis in the United States: still room for improvement. *Journal of General Internal Medicine,* Vol 25, No. 6 (June), pp. 484-486, ISSN 0884-8734

Stewart, G.J.; Ritchie, W.G. & Lynch, P.R. (1974). Venous endothelial damage produced by massive sticking and emigration of leukocytes. *American Journal of Pathology,* Vol. 74, No. 3 (March), pp. 507-532, ISSN 0002-9440

Talbott, J.H. (1970). *A Biographical History of Medicine: Excerpts and Essays on the Men and their Work.* Grune and Stratton, New York

Ten, V.S. & Pinsky, D.J. (2002). Endothelial response to hypoxia: physiologic adaptation and pathologic dysfunction. *Current Opinion in Critical Care,* Vol. 8, No. 3 (June), pp. 242-250, ISSN 1070-5295

Thiagarajan, P. (2002). New targets for antithrombotic drugs. *American Journal of Cardiovascular Drugs,* Vol. 2, No. 4, pp. 227-235, ISSN 1175-3277

Thomas, D.P. (1988). Overview of venous thrombogenesis. *Seminars in Thrombosis and Hemostasis,* Vol. 14, No. 1 (January), pp. 1-8, ISSN 0094-6176

Trotman, W.E.; Taatjes, D.J.; Callas, P.W. & Bovill, E.G. (2011). The endothelial microenvironment in the venous valvular sinus: thromboresistance trends and inter-individual variation. *Histochemistry and Cell Biology,* Vol. 135, No. 2 (February), pp. 141-152, ISSN 0948-6143

Van Langevelde, K.; Sramek, A. & Rosendaal, F.R. (2010). The effect of ageing on venous valves. *Arteriosclerosis, Thrombosis, and Vascular Biology,* Vol. 30, No. 10 (October), pp. 275–80, ISSN 1079-5642

Van Ottingen, W.F. (1941). *Studies on the Mechanism of Carbon Monoxide Poisoning as Observed in Dogs Anesthetized with Sodium Amytal.* United States Public Health Service, Washington DC

Virchow, R.L.K. (1856). *Thrombosis und Embolie.* In *Klassiker der Medizin herausgegeben von Karl Sudhoff,* Barth, J.A. (ed.) Leipzig (1910). Translated by Matzdorff, A.C. & Bell, W.R. (1998). Science History Publications, ISBN 0-88135-113-X, Canton

Virchow, R.L.K. (1858). *Die Cellularpathologie in ihrer Begründung auf physiologische und pathologische Gewebelehre.* A. Hirschwald, Berlin

Virchow, R.L.K. (1862). *Gessamelte Abhandlungen zur wissenschaftlichen Medizin von Rudolf Virchow.* Meidinger, Frankfurt am Main

Welch, W.H. (1887). The structure of white thrombi. *Transactions of the Pathological Society of Philadelphia,* Vol. 13, pp. 281-300

Welch, W.H. (1899). Thrombosis, In *A System of Medicine,* vol. 6, Allbutt, C. (ed.), pp. 155-165, Macmillan, London

Wessler, S. (1962). Thrombosis in the presence of vascular stasis. *American Journal of Medicine,* Vol. 33 (November), pp. 648–666, ISSN 0002-9343

Wright, H.P. & Osborn, S.B. (1952). Venous velocity in bedridden medical patients. *Lancet,* Vol. 2, No. 6737 (October), pp. 699-700, ISSN 0140-6736

Yan, S.-F.; Mackman, N.; Kisiel, W.; Stern, D.M. & Pinsky, D.J. (1999a). Hypoxia/hypoxemia-induced activation of the procoagulant pathways and the pathogenesis of ischemia-associated thrombosis. *Arteriosclerosis, Thrombosis, and Vascular Biology,* Vol. 19, No. 9 (September), pp. 2029-2035, ISSN 1079-5642

Yan, S.-F.; Lu, J.; Zou, Y.S.; Soh-Won, J.; Cohen, D.M.; Buttrick, P.M.; Cooper, D.R.; Steinberg, S.F.; Mackman, N.; Pinsky, D.J. & Stern, D.M. (1999b). Hypoxia-associated induction of early growth response-1 gene expression. *The Journal of Biological Chemistry,* Vol. 274, No. 21 (May), pp. 15030-15040, ISSN 0021-9258

Zahn, F.W. (1876). Untersuchungen über Thrombose. *Zentralblatt für den medizinische Wissenschaft,* Vol. 10, pp. 129-153

Zweifach, B.W. (1963). Peripheral vascular factors in the genesis of stasis and thrombosis. *Federation Proceedings,* Vol. 22 (November-December), pp. 1351-1355, ISSN 0014-9446

7

Venous Thromboembolism as a Preventable Patient Injury: Experience of the Danish Patient Insurance Association (1996 - 2010)

Jens Krogh Christoffersen[1] and Lars Dahlgaard Hove[2]
[1]*Danish Patient Insurance Association,*
[2]*Hvidovre Hospital, University of Copenhagen,*
Denmark

1. Introduction

The mechanism of disease in venous thromboembolsm (VTE) is mentioned, with emphasis on the rarer types of the disease. Next the conditions for approval of claims under the Danish Patient Insurance law are drawn up, and the typical situations for approval of VTE are listed. In the database of the DPIA we found 688 claims with this disease, and of these 421 were approved. The different types of VTE are examined, and the possibilities for prevention are discussed.

2. Of venous thromboembolism

Venous trombosis is usually located in the veins of the lower extremity. The thrombosis probably has its origin in the valve pockets of the veins of the lower leg. There are several pathogenetic factors, but a common denominator is reduction of flow velocity in the veins. This may occur in a varity of situations, e.g.:

1. During aneasthesia it has been shown that the diameter of the veins increase, and thus the velocity of the flow decreases. At the same time the operative trauma increases the readyness of the thrombotic system.
2. In a number of different trauma situations to the leg, where immobilisation in casts or splints is used, rendering the venous muscle pump dysfunctionate,
3. In acute stroke, the afflicted leg is left without its normal venous muscle pump

These are classic examples of patients that may suffer a deep venous trombosis (DVT) or more severely a pumonary embolism (PE).

There are many clinical examples of variatons on the theme.

The thrombosis may begin in the popliteal or femoral vein progressing centrally until it breaks off and sends its potentially fatal embolism to the lungs. It may also have its origin in the iliac veins, in which case the diameter of the ensuing embolism is sufficient large to close off the entire pulmonary artery, causing immediate death.

A special variety of the disease exists, where an obstruction is present at the iliac venous junction. This is called the *left iliac vein syndrome,* and it is normally not associated with pulmonary embolism, as the lumen of the left common vena iliaca is partially obstructed by a fine net of the endothelium at the junction. The compression from the crossing of the right common iliac artery adds to the obstruction.

In some cases the source of embolism is located in a venous malformation, and the thrombi to the lungs may be small and not easily clinically detectable. The pressure in the pulmonary artery increases slowly over months with the continuing pulmonal embolization causing cronical *cor pulmonale.* The *foramen ovale* may open under the increased pressure in the right side of the heart, releasing minor emboli to the arterial circulation. The end result is usually cardiac arrest due to the increased pressure with dilation of the right ventricle.

In rare cases the thrombosis occurs in the veins of the upper extremity. The size of emboli from the arms is not sufficient to give any serious problem from the lungs, but it is important to know that this possibility exists.

Thombosis in the mesenteric veins is a very rare, but potentially deadly disease. The onset of symptoms is much slower than that of arterial vascular iscaemia, where as a rule you have only 6 hours from the embolization to completion of thrombectomy, if gangrene and resection should be prevented. In venous ishaemia there are often days or weeks of symptoms before the onset of gangrene, and if the ischaemia has progressed to gangrene, a simple resection will often be sufficient. Venous intestinal ischaemia is usually not recognized until laparotomy, and it may be very difficult to make the diagnosis by laparoscopy alone.

Thrombosis in the venous sinuses of the brain is an important side effect to birth control drugs, and must always be considered as a differential diagnosis when a patient on the pill develops symptoms from the brain.

Finally, another inborn vascular anomaly has bearing on the embolisation from the veins of the lower limbs: The *foramen ovale,* which normally closes at the time of birth, will sometimes remain open and allow emboli from the right side to cross over to the left side and continue in the arterial system. This is known as "paradox" embolisation, and is important to consider, when a patient at risk for venous thrombosis suffers an arterial embolus. The frequency of patent *foramen ovale* in autopsy studies is about 20 %, so this a significant risk, as the frequency of deep venous thrombosis is equally high (1).

The disease known as thrombophlebitis, where a subcutaneous vein is inflamed and thrombosed, has nothing in common with DVT. In the major part of the 20th century it was thought that thrombosis might spread from the superficial veins to the femoral venous system through the sapheno-femoral junction, wherefore acute ligature of the junction was advised. This indication for the sapheno-femoral ligature has since been abandoned. Also, the practice of anticoagulation with thrombophlebitis is no longer advised.

3. The Danish patient insurance law

In Denmark, patients or relatives may file a claim if their medical treatment results in an injury or an unexpected side effect. The independent Danish Patient Insurance

Association (DPIA) will consider these claims. The DPIA operates on a no-blame, no-fault basis and does not take any legal action beyond assessing damages. As a result, patients may file a claim with the DPIA free of charge with the sole purpose of seeking financial compensation. Thus, the injured patient is spared the expense of legal fees and the trouble of going to court (2).

In general, financial compensation may be granted under any one of the following conditions:

1. an experienced specialist would have acted differently, whereby the injury would have been avoided,
2. defects in or failure of the technical equipment were of major concern with respect to the incident,
3. the injury could have been avoided by using alternative treatments, techniques or methods if these were considered to be equally safe and potentially offer the same benefits, and finally,
4. the injury is rare, serious, and more extensive than the patient should be expected to endure.

Compensation is calculated based on the extent of pain and suffering, reduced income, reduced ability to work, and medical expenses as well as whether the injury could be expected to be permanent. Compensation is rendered if the calculated amount exceeds 1,500 €. The government pays the compensations. After the decision has been made, the patient may file an appeal to the Patient Damage Appeal Board and further through the courts of law. From 1996 to 2010, the DPIA received 64.400 claims; 34.9 % of these were approved.

4. Venous tromboembolism and patient injury

VTE may be judged to be a patient injury in the following situations:

- when an injury was sustained, because the diagnosis of VTE was not made in a situation, where an experienced specialist would have done so,
- when VTE has been caused by giving a treament wthout the proper prophylaxis,
- when a drug was prescribed that caused VTE,
- when the treatment of VTE was not up to the standard of the experienced specialist
- when the patient suffered more than he should be expected to bear considering his basic disease, the risk of treatment and whether the complication was rare and serious.

In such cases the DPIA may consider to give compensation if the other conditions of the law are met.

5. VTE and the database of the DPIA

Since 1996 we have maintained a database of all claims. Until the end of 2010, there were 688 claims, where the complication was VTE. In table 1 is shown the number of patients with DVT alone, the patients who also had PE, and the patients with rare thombosis. The rates of approval of the claims are around 60 % compared to the average rate of 35 % of the DPIA.

Complication	N	N approved	Rate of approval
Deep venous thrombosis in the legs alone	390	226	58 %
Pulmonary embolism	266	176	66 %
Rare venous thrombosis	32	19	59 %
Total	688	421	61 %

Table 1. DVT and PE in the material.

There were 42 patients who died because of the patient injury (6.1 %).

The patients could be divided in 5 sub-categories after the nature of their disease and circumstances surrounding the injury (Table 2).

Invasive procedures	391
Birth control drugs	193
Other drugs	13
Non-operative fracture treatment	30
Missed diagnosis	15
Rare and miscellaneus	46
Total	688

Table 2. Categories of patients.

VTE after an open intervention was the largest group with 391 patients. The cause of injury was usually failing to give the correct prophylaxis, or omitting to give any prophylaxis at all. The specialities involved are seen in table 3.

Speciality	N invasive procedures	N approved
Orthopedic surgery	226	128
Surgery	94	52
Internal medicine	23	10
Gynaecology & Obstetrics	18	11
Neurosurgery	13	9
General practice	2	2
OtoRhinoLaryngology	5	5
Anaestesia	3	2
Radiology	4	3
Neurology	1	1
Onchology	1	0
Dental surgery	1	1
Total	391	224

Table 3. The number of patients with VTE treated in the different specialities.

Of these, 27 patients died as result of the injury. There were 224 patients, who had their claims approved by the DPIA. Compensation was paid to 218 patients to the total amount of € 6.127.365.

6. VTE and treatment with female hormones

The other large group was 193 patients with DVT or PE, who had birth control medication (173 patients) or treatment of menopausal conditions (20 patients) prescribed by their physician, and suffered VTE as a result. Their claims were approved in 138 cases, and € 2.956.248 was paid to 134 patients. Only 5 women died, but it must be borne in mind that these were completely healthy women. In 17 cases it was later established that the patient had a coagulation defect, usually the Leiden factor-5 mutation.

There were at times several factors that contributed to the onset of thrombosis in these patients. Thus it was discussed which factor was the crucial one, when e.g. a young woman who was on birth control pills and had a body mass index of 34, undertook a long air travel and suffered VTE? The coagulation experts that we have consulted thought that the VTE would not have happened without the birth control medication, and that the contribution of the other factors was minor in comparison.

7. Treatment with other drugs

In 12 cases the VTE was thought to be caused by other drugs (Table 4). It was mainly claims with faulty use of anticoagulants that were approved. One patient died.

Other drugs	N	N approved
Vitamin K antagonist	5	3
Angiotensin converting enzyme	1	1
Immuneglobuline	2	1
Docetaxel	3	0
Cox-2 inhibitor	1	0
Prednisolone	1	0
	13	5

Table 4. The other drugs involved in VTE claims.

Non-operative treatment of fractures and joint injuries was the cause of 30 claims, shown in table 5.

Non-operative treatment of fractures and joint injuries	N	N approved
Spine	3	1
Lower extremity	27	13
	30	14

Table 5. VTE after non-operative treatment.

It was of course mainly fractures in the lower extremity that were afflicted because of the need for immobilization. Usually in the DPIA, VTE is thought to be a side effect of the fracture itself, and it is therefore not eligible for compensation. In 4 cases however, the diagnosis was missed, and in one further case the appeal board decided that the diagnosis should have been made at the time, when the cast was cut open because of swelling. In the last 9 approved cases there were individual indications for giving anticoagulants that were not recognized at the time of fracture. Four patients died as a result of the patient injury. In many of the non-approved cases, the question was whether the experienced specialist would have used prophylaxis? For example, the recommended program for a non-displaced fracture of the tibia states that prophylaxis against VTE is not necessary; yet the frequency of DVT in these patients is 15 %. If we were to extend the program of prophylaxis to encompass ambulatory patients with a walking cast, these patients would only rarely suffer DVT, and some lives would be spared.

8. Missed diagnosis

In 15 cases without fractures or operation, the diagnosis of VTE was missed. The claim was approved in 12 cases (Table 6). These cases were evenly distributed among primary and secondary practice. Three patients died as result of the injury

	N	Approved
Hospitals	7	6
Primary sector	8	6
	15	12

Table 6. The number of missed or overlooked diagnosis of VTE.

9. Miscellaneous

The remaining 45 cases were a broad selection of the many different causes there may be for acquiring VTE, as well as a few that had a prophylaxis or a treatment of VTE that wasn't up to the standard of the experienced specialist (Table 7).

Rare or miscellaneous	N	N approved
Upper extremity	20	10
Sinus thrombosis	11	9
Venous puncture or catheterization	4	4
Wrong prophylaxis or treatment	4	4
VTE i spite of correct treatment	3	0
Mesenteric venous thrombosis	2	1
Paradox embolism	1	1
	45	29

Table 7. Rare or miscelleanous patients.

The cases of cerebral sinus thrombosis were all caused by birth control medication. Three of the cases of venous puncture were caused by blood donation; such claims are nearly always approved by the DPIA. Two of the 45 patients died.

There were 83 claims that went on to the appeal board, and of these 15 had the decision of the DPIA altered. The changes of decisions nearly all concerned the size of the compensation. One claim went on to the high court. It concerned a male of 33 years, who had a percutaneous endoscopic ligature of the spermatic veins for a *hydrocele testis*. Afterwards he suffered a hemorrhage in the scrotal sac and a venous thrombosis in the leg. The compensation in the DPIA was € 95.165, and this decision was upheld both before the appeal board and in the high court.

10. Discussion

The standard prophylaxis in Denmark is usually given only for the duration of admittance to hospital, or until the patient is well mobilized. During recent times, a number of studies have suggested that this is not enough, and that prophylaxis should be given for 6 or 8 weeks after surgery (3, 4). The price would be manageable, and the logistics could probably be overcome. Why do we accept that hundreds and hundreds of patients go without prophylaxis for the period they are at risk?

Also, it is not rare to see a patient described as "well mobilized" and therefore have his prophylaxis discontinued, when in fact he is only out of bed for a few hours a day and then only sitting in a chair. The sitting position, if anything, increases the stasis of blood in the veins of the legs, and therefore probably also increases the risk of VTE. The development of tablets for VTE prophylaxis may change this state of affairs in the future, since it will make the administration of medication simpler (5, 6).

The treatment of VTE goes hand in hand with the prevention of the disease. When you have seen the damage that VTE can do to patients, you are likely to go far to prevent a single case. There exists well-proven mechanical as well as biochemical methods with very few side effects. All of these 688 cases must be viewed as potentially preventable with the exception of the 3 cases, where VTA occurred in spite of the fact that correct prophylaxis was given. Off course it is not possible to prevent all cases, which you can se by the fact that these 3 cases occurred. But this must not be given as an excuse to omit prophylaxis.

It is inexcusable to perform major invasive treatment without prophylaxis, and probably the medical profession should consider extending the indications as well as the duration of prophylaxis. The cost of doing this will be balanced against the gain from not having to treat the VTE-cases and the tax returns from the survivors of complications to VTE (7).

It should probably also be considered to screen the women for coagulation deficits before they are placed on contraceptive medication. Certainly, it is clear from our records, that the medical profession should consider the differential diagnosis of VTE in patients on contraceptive drugs more often.

For the DPIA it is also a question whether you should approve claims from women, who have a coagulation defect like Leiden factor-5 mutation? There were only 17 cases where our patients had been tested positive for this genetic defect. The true number is probably much higher. Normally, the DPIA does not approve claims, when a patient has a disposition to the injury. It can be argued, however, that the experienced specialist would not prescribe contraceptive drugs to a patient with Leiden-5 mutation. It is therefore the normal practice of the DPIA to approve these claims.

The fractures that are treated by non-invasive means are by no means immune from VTE. A recent metaanalysis of the question of prophylaxis to these patients (8) states that ambulatory patients with temporary lower leg immobilization who are over 50, in a rigid cast, non-weight bearing or with a severe injury should be considered as a risk group for VTE. The present opinion is however, that the VTE in these cases is caused by the trauma and not the treatment. The patient that dies from PE probably doesn't care. We think that it should be seriously considered to include these patients in an anti-VTE program.

We realize that there are many claims that never comes to the knowledge of the DPIA. The reasons for this are many: Ignorance of the law, resignation in the face of a serious disease complicated by the injury, the bother of the application procedure, fear of alienating the physician etc. We have tried several methods in order to achieve a more precise estimate of this problem (9, 10). Our best estimate is now that there are at least 4 - 5 patient injuries for each claim.

The risk of VTE increases with malignancy, infections, reoperations and surgery close to the large veins. The prophylaxis should be adjusted accordingly. It is about time that the medical profession starts to realize that posttraumatic or postoperative VTE is not an inevitable event. It may be prevented by a number of quite effective measures, but a change in attitude from the medical profession is required.

11. References

[1] Brownwall E. Textbook of Cardiology p. 985. WB Saunders, Philadelphia 1988

[2] http://www.patientforsikringen.dk/en/Love-og-Regler.aspx.

[3] Bottaro FJ, Elizondo MC, Doti C, Bruetman JE, Perez Moreno PD, Bullorsky EO,Ceresetto JM. Efficacy of extended thrombo-prophylaxis in major abdominalsurgery: what does the evidence show? A meta-analysis. Thromb Haemost. 2008;99(6):1104-11.

[4] Rasmussen MS, Jorgensen LN, Wille-Jørgensen P, Nielsen JD, Horn A, Mohn AC,Sømod L, Olsen B; FAME Investigators. Prolonged prophylaxis with dalteparin to prevent late thromboembolic complications in patients undergoing major abdominal surgery: a multicenter randomized open-label study. J Thromb Haemost. 2006;4(11):2384-90.

[5] Schulman S, Majeed A. A benefit-risk assessment of dabigatran in the prevention of venous thromboembolism in orthopaedic surgery. Drug Saf. 2011;34(6):449-63.

[6] Bovio JA, Smith SM, Gums JG. Dabigatran etexilate: a novel oral thrombin inhibitor for thromboembolic disease. Ann Pharmacother. 2011;45(5):603-14.)

[7] Ruppert A, Steinle T, Lees M. Economic burden of venous thromboembolism: asystematic review. J Med Econ. 2011;14(1):65-74.

[8] No authors listed. Evidence exists to guide thromboembolic prophylaxis in ambulatory patients with temporary lower limb immobilisation. Emerg Med J. 2011;28(8):718-20.

[9] Erichsen M, Rasmussen CW, Christoffersen JK. Pulmonary embolism with lethal outcome and claims to the Danish Patient Insurance Association. Ugeskr læg 2008; 170(22): 1909-1912

[10] Petersen HØ, Rasmussen AH, Andersen LI, Christoffersen JK. Mediastinitis following cardiac surgery. Patient insurance reports. Ugeskrift for læger 2008; 170(22): 1907-1908,

Made in the USA
Las Vegas, NV
15 November 2026

fa339ba1-b7dc-41dc-abee-30ec62d87cc0R01